My Broken Heart

Conquering Heart Disease

By Rochelle Bos

ISBN: 1983935999
ISBN-13: 978-1983935992

Hope? Or Despair?

Room 28-B. At least I had the bed by the window to view the stark snowless landscape of the late fall. The white-board on the bland hospital wall, with the name of my nurse, indicated my mobility status as "independent". How long would that last? If I were to ever see the outside world again, would I still be independent, or an invalid? Wheelchair? Oxygen? Walker? Which would be worse – revisiting the world with limited capacity to enjoy it, or never seeing the world or my family again, or they seeing me? Doubts, fears, anxiety. The repulsive hospital odors and sounds did nothing to improve my optimism, which normally was quite high.

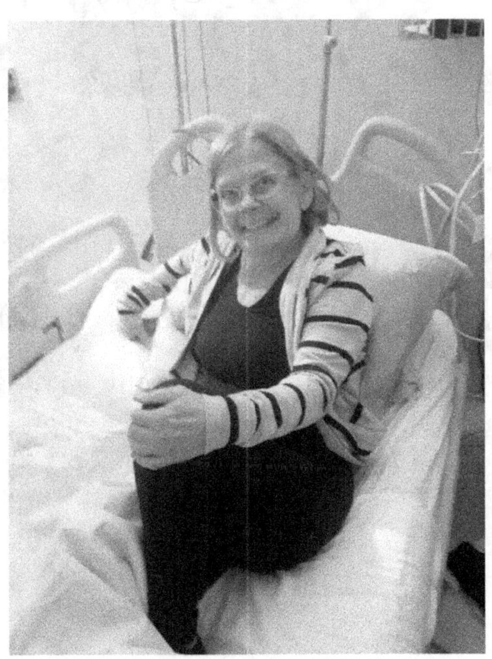

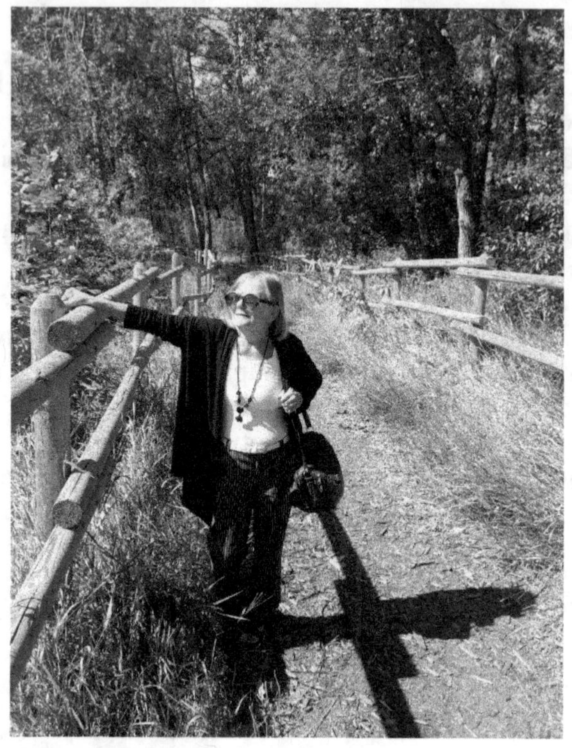

The mild weather of late fall/early winter had made my last months of "independence" a treasure. Long walks by the river with Brian. I even had a final road trip to see my precious Anika who was now 2 ½ years old. I prayed - no that's silly, I don't pray – that I would see her again and hear her laughter and newly found and growing vocabulary. Lori took me on a girls' weekend to the mountains the week prior to admission.

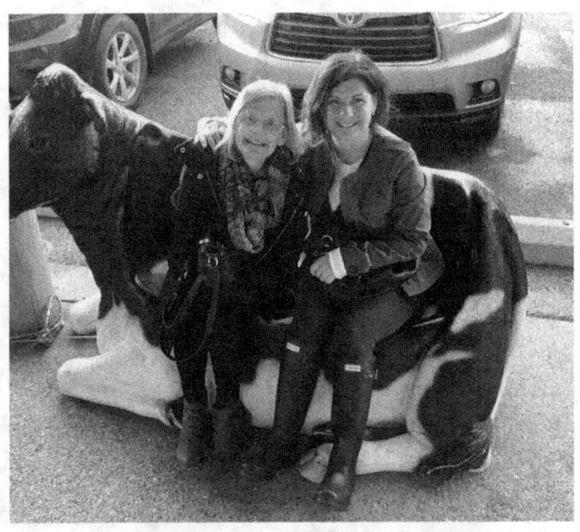

The day before my admission was a mixed blessing. I had a chance to visit with Lori, Rob and their families, but I felt compelled to give the "what-if" talk." What if I didn't make it? Grant assured me I would make it – he had found a "lucky" penny he was keeping in his shoe until my return.

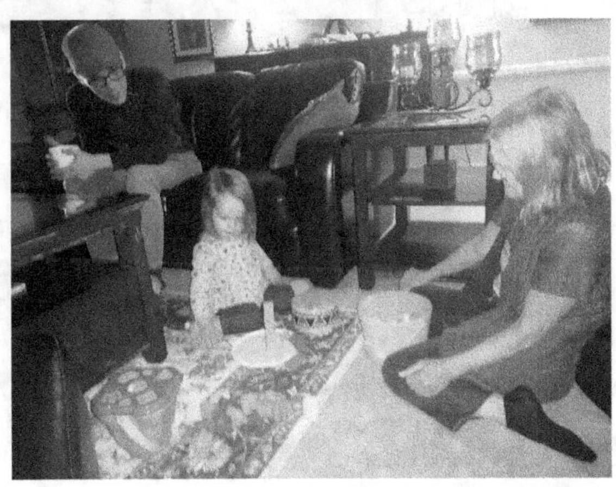

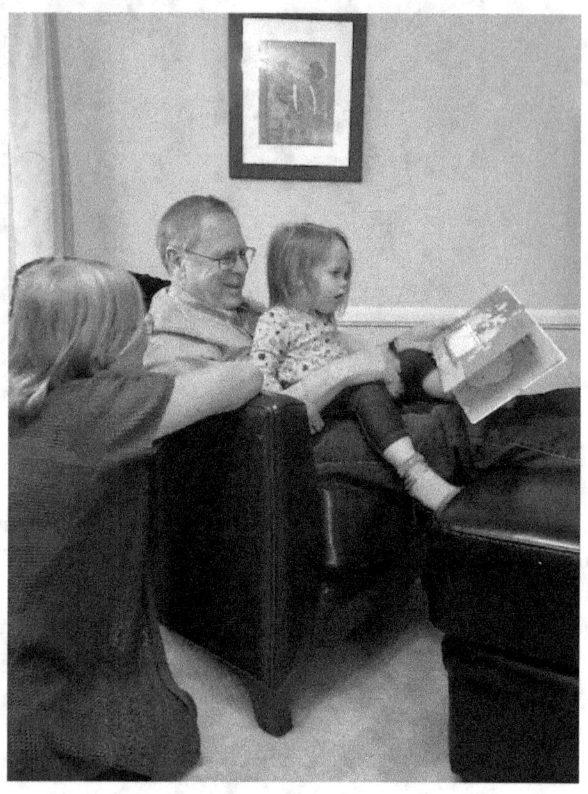

This was to be my "hat trick", my third time (or was it to be three strikes and you're out). As such, my chances of surviving the operation were reduced considerably. Some surgeons, looking at the 30% probability of failure, refused to consider my case. However, Doctor Kidd felt he could reduce the risk to 10% - better, but still not great. A one in ten chance I would never see another day.

Would this time be more like my easy-peasy first time, or like the disaster of my second? I had two days left to toss all of these thoughts around in my mind, which was in constant turmoil. At least my "independent" status allowed me the freedom to visit freely with Lori, Rob and their families in the coffee shop or cafeteria. Brian chased Anika around the hospital corridors; even in my current healthy state, I could not keep up with the active toddler. Rob and Annaliese had continued to keep my spirits up by sending daily videos of Anika being Anika. Lori, after one of our lunches before the operation. said, "You know, Mom, what you said at your last operation? You said 'I'm not going anywhere, people need me, I've things to do'. Nothing has changed, we all still need you and you still have things to do." She was right – I hoped.

The First Time - 1981

I barely remember the first time; in retrospect it seems like such a non-event. My late husband, Chris and I decided that the operation was so routine that he should use this opportunity over the summer, to take our two young children, Lori and Rob, to see Chris' dying mother in Holland. I was home recuperating by the time they returned from their trip, and back teaching by the end of the summer.

I was born with a broken heart - a murmur they called it at the time. The left ventricle of the heart pumps the blood through the aorta and the aortic valve opens to let the blood through, but closes to prevent the blood from returning the left ventricle when it relaxes. My aortic valve leaked, allowing some blood to leak back into the left ventricle.

The post-World War II era gave rise the "baby-boomers" of which I was one. The few of us who were born with such a heart condition just had to live with it - or die with it, in some cases. It was a condition that could be diagnosed, but not treated. Families with money or inclination might be able to get doctors to help such children, but my parents had neither money nor inclination. They were the "go-along to get-along" type. They quietly accepted whatever cards they were dealt and kept them close to their chest.

I was small in stature, likely because of my heart condition, and my parents just tried to keep me out of sight. They acted as if they were ashamed of me, or at least they never displayed any pride in their only offspring. I was considered a sickly child and treated as such. My parents never gave me any praise or guidance - they just tolerated my existence. It was important to my parents that they be seen as upright and proper, and I did not contribute to their needs. I reacted, or retaliated with a stubborn streak with a tinge of rebelliousness. Not so much when I was young, but definitely when I reached my teens. I refused to be held back by my condition, nor by my stoic, plastic parents. One benefit of my heart ailment was that I never had to attend gym class – I was completely un-athletic and hated gym class.

I was acutely aware of my heart condition, which was made clear to me often enough by my parents. As a result, my rebelliousness did not extend to the behaviours of other teens of the sixties. I chose not to drink alcohol, I chose not to smoke cigarettes and I stayed away from the drug scene that was so prevalent at the time. These behaviours were all around me, but I was able to navigate through them unaffected. It probably helped that I was part of the "geek" crowd, and therefore not pressured to comply with the "cool" kids. I was short and often referred to as "cute", but was relegated to the less than attractive groups.

I rebelled in other ways, such as dating boys who were not of a standard acceptable to my parents. Appearance meant everything to them and my appearance was often a source of embarrassment for them - especially my choice of partners. I couldn't wait to get away from my parents and their disapproving eye. But as a low achiever with limited appeal I had minimal opportunities to escape. My father convinced me to take a traditional "woman's" job as a secretary and pushed me to a business college where I achieved limited success. To help support my efforts, I worked as a hippie waitress in a coffee house that featured upcoming folk singers. Another point of rebellion.

I wanted to go to a real university and get a real job. I saved my pennies, took out student loans and went to university to get a two-year teaching certificate. With that parchment in hand, I was able to escape my parents and their city. I moved to Calgary where I taught elementary school.

The rebel that had emerged in me continued beyond the scope of my parents. When one particular boyfriend was tardy in presenting me with a marriage proposal, I dumped him and picked up a soldier in a bar. Within months, I married the soldier and moved to a British Columbia lower mainland Canadian Forces base, where I became a teacher for the children of the services members. My status as a teacher gave me officer privileges that exceeded those of the enlisted man status of my new husband. I wasn't very kind to him and constantly berated him for his lowly status. So, it was no surprise when our marriage began to show some signs of disrepair.

We never discussed having a family, but I became pregnant. I looked forward to having a baby to care for and thought this may be a way to save my failing marriage. When doctors determined I was having a baby, they became concerned that my heart condition may not allow me to carry a baby to term. Through a series of tests, they found that my heart would likely survive giving birth and permitted me to carry my baby. But they refused to let me have a natural birth and insisted on a caesarean delivery. Late in the year, Lori emerged to brighten my life; my heart survived but my marriage did not. I reluctantly told my mother that I was leaving my marriage, due to my husband's infidelity and she instructed me to return to my marriage and "be a better wife - try harder." I rebelled again; Lori and I struck out on our own.

I met and married Chris a few years later. He embraced our ready-made family and my faulty heart. I became pregnant a second time, and my heart was just strong enough to allow me to bring Robert into the world - again by caesarean delivery. But by now, my heart murmur was accelerating, threatening my long-term survival.

In the over thirty years since my heart condition was recognized, the medical profession had advanced to the point where there were now fixes for my congenital problem. One option was installing an artificial aortic valve. As I was still of child-bearing age and still having my periods, the doctors advised against an artificial valve. Having such a valve would require that I go on blood thinners, making me susceptible to fatal bleeding. Instead, they opted for transplanting the heart valve from a pig. The doctors informed me that this was only a temporary solution until I was past having my period. The operation was fairly routine and I was back to work within six weeks of having my chest split and heart opened to install the new valve. I was never a vain person, but bikinis were now banned from my wardrobe as I had a telltale scar down the middle of my chest to match the scars from my two caesarean births.

No guarantees, but my new valve was to last a dozen years. It was actually closer to fifteen years before my pig valve began to show signs of failure.

Round Two - 1997

The doctors told me that my aortic valve (pig valve) had reached the end of its life and was going to fail completely. Given that I was now fifty years old and had a hysterectomy a few years ago, it was best that I replace it with an artificial valve as I could now take blood thinners (warfarin or coumadin). It was supposed to be a routine operation, much like the last one over fifteen years earlier. One time digging into the heart is fairly low risk; a second time provides an increased risk; but the risk of not doing the operation was higher than the risk of doing it. So, I agreed - living was a better option than not living. Chris, Rob and Lori took this operation more seriously than the first one and stayed close to home for my support. The plan was for a spring operation, recovery over the summer and back to teaching in the fall. Looking back, this is actually what happened, but there were a few detours along the way.

The trip into the operating room felt familiar, as it mirrored my experience from fifteen years prior. The initial drugs made me calm and sedate, almost giddy - but confident. By the time I hit the operating room, I was oblivious to anything around me.

My next memory was of being encased in cement - or so I thought. I could not move any part of my body; it was frozen. My eyes would not open; I could not see anything. But I could think; my mind was fully functional, and I could hear. That was the scariest part - I could HEAR. I could hear everything that was going on around me. I could fully understand the words that were spoken by nurses and by doctors and by Chris. I could detect the tone and the severity of those speaking; but I could not respond - neither by speaking nor by motion. I was in an induced coma - my body could not function; however, my brain and ears did. My brain processed the pieces of data that entered my ears. Some of the sounds were whispers, but most were loud enough to absorb and interpret.

My operation had not gone well - a bit of an understatement. My acute hearing and alert mind helped me piece together what had happened and what was happening now.

With my sternum pulled apart to expose my heart, removal of the pig valve was more of a challenge than anticipated. The pig skin had fused to my heart muscle creating scar tissue. Pulling the pig skin from my heart caused damage to my heart. The doctors installed my new artificial aortic valve on my damaged heart thinking that everything would be OK. They closed my chest and began wheeling me to the Intensive Care Unit, with my body attached to a variety of wires, tubes and monitoring equipment. Going into the ICU, all of the monitors began to shout warning signals - I was bleeding inside my chest, bleeding to death. They rushed me back to the operating room where they reopened my chest to locate the source of the bleeding - it was a mess, the bleeding seemed to be coming from everywhere. They couldn't fully stop the bleeding, so they packed my chest with material to impede the bleeding and pushed me into the Intensive Care Unit with my body frozen and my chest wide open. The doctors needed to develop a plan of action - or inaction.

After I had mentally processed my predicament, I tuned my ears to capture every sound emanating from the medical professionals that hovered around my still body. One particular exchange put my predicament into perspective and forced me to develop my own plan of attack.

"You had better call in the family," a doctor told Chris. "I doubt she will make it through the night."

I felt my body shiver at this revelation, but my body couldn't actually shiver. So, it was my mind that felt cold.

"*Wait a minute*," my mind shouted in silence. "*I'm not going anywhere*." I resolved to overrule the doctor's prognostication. I was going to make it through this, in spite of my frail and failing body. I turned to visualization.

I started small, by picturing myself in a regular hospital room attached to my intravenous pole. In my mind, I stood up and began walking up and down the hospital hallway. Once I had mastered that exercise, I began mentally walking into my back yard. I sat in a lawn chair soaking up the warm sun while listening to the trickling pond that Chris had installed. I then insisted on taking a vacation to Europe to visit Holland, France and Spain. The south of Spain was especially comforting to the rehabilitation that was transpiring in my mind.

My mental journey, over the five days I was in a comatose state with my chest laying open, was often interrupted by the mundane conversations among employees in the ICU. I knew when a nurse was having marital problems. I found out who was having pizza for supper and who was having steak. These many interruptions to my mental gyrations were just annoying distractions and didn't keep me from my ultimate mission.

Chris sat by my side speaking as though he knew I could hear, "I need you, the kids need you." I recall Lori crying beside my bed, while being comforted by a friend.

By the fifth day as a bodiless being, the doctors had stemmed the bleeding and I was taken back for the final closure of my chest. They determined that my heart would no longer work on its own after the trauma it had undergone. I was outfitted with a Pacemaker connected to a wire lead into my heart through the tricuspid valve. The lead connected to a generator (battery) installed under the skin below my right shoulder on my chest, and an emergency lead that created an unsightly bump below my breastbone. I was set for my recovery - the most memorable event after awaking was having Rob spoon some ice chips to the back of my tongue. I have loved ice ever since. Lori was there to see my first "thumbs-up" gesture.

With the help and support of Chris, Lori and Rob, I walked out of the hospital and spent time in my backyard as I had visualized. Chris took me on our European vacation that summer, including time in the south of Spain. By that fall I was back teaching my grade two students.

The sad irony of my near-death experience is that I lost Chris to cancer barely two years after my miraculous recovery.

Blowing the Pacemaker

Given my small stature, I was never athletic. However, with Chris' prompting, I became a recreational runner. My fitness level before my second operation was likely a contributing factor to my recovery. After regaining my strength, I returned to running, even competing (competing may be an overstatement) in short road races. On one such 5-km race I found my energy completely sapped, long before I reached the finish line. I could barely keep up a slow walk as I returned to my car, skipping the post race festivities. Chris had uncharacteristically stayed home from the race, claiming to feel poorly. What a wimp - I was the one who nearly died from heart surgery. Looking back, this was one of the first signs that Chris was entering the final months of his life.

I told Chris of my problem when I got home from the race and we scooted to the hospital emergency to see what my problem was - I still hadn't regained my ability to move beyond a slow shuffle. It didn't take long for the hospital staff to discover the source of my difficulty - it was my Pacemaker. When the Pacemaker was installed in my body, the settings used were similar to those they would give any sedentary senior citizen. But I was neither a senior citizen, nor was I sedentary. The Pacemaker had a lower limit of 60 beats per minute and an upper limit of 120 beats per minute - a sensible setting for most heart patients. If your heart rate exceeds the upper limit, the assumption is that you are having a heart attack and the Pacemaker has an emergency mode that resets to a constant 60 beats per minute. At this heart rate a person can function at a low level until they receive medical attention. In my case, my racing had pushed my heart rate above the upper limit and the Pacemaker reset, making all but limited movement impossible. All the Pacemaker technician had to do was to wave a magic wand over my chest, just like in Star Trek, and restore my original settings.

I insisted that they give me more capacity due to my ability to push my heart beyond that of a sedentary old lady. They complied with an upper setting of 150 beats per minute and I continued my "racing career".

After Chris' death, I decided to take Lori and Rob to visit Chris' family in Holland, and take in some European history and culture. With a couple of years of experience with my Pacemaker, I knew enough not to go through the metal detectors at airports or I would face the same fate as in the race. In Greece, Lori developed food poisoning and stayed in the hotel room while Rob and I explored. In addition to visiting some of the ancient sites, we stopped into various galleries and book stores. Upon entering one particular store, we went from the hot humid air of the outside, to the cool air of the store, and I fell to the floor in a faint. Poor Rob had just lost his father and now his mother lay unconscious on the floor in a foreign country. I came around fairly quickly and we at first assumed that I had just fainted due to the rapid change in temperature. But as I started to move around I knew what was wrong. I was experiencing the same sensations I had when I crashed during my race. The security detector at the door, where we entered, had set off my Pacemaker.

That meant I was stuck with a heart rate of 60 beats per minute until I could locate a Pacemaker technician with a magic wand. A quick read of our travel guide convinced us that one of the last places in the world you wanted to visit a medical facility was Greece. Lori stayed in Greece to catch up on the exploring she had missed, while Rob took his doddering old mother on to Rome.

In Rome we made our first stop the hospital where language was a major barrier. As the doctors checked me over they determined I was OK and wanted to send me on my way. Try as I might I could not convince them of my plight. We were able to make contact with the Pacemaker people back in Canada and when they heard that our next stop was Amsterdam, they instructed me to contact their office in that city - my particular device had actually been manufactured at the Medtronic's plant in that city. So, I shuffled through the rest of our side trip and waited for Holland.

Once in Holland, Chris' brother was quite helpful in putting us in touch with the Medtronic's office. A technician met us, carrying his fully equipped briefcase, waved his magic wand over my chest and I was cured.

I made the obligatory trip to the Pacemaker clinic when we returned to Canada. The Pacemaker doctor and technician chuckled at having followed my adventures in Europe after my incident. They were able to track my movements across the continent.

I made frequent visits to the University library back home, but was very careful not to go near the theft detectors. In spite of my caution, I set off my

Pacemaker several times, requiring trips to the Pacemaker clinic to be cured by the magic wand. After the third such trip, I asked for a better solution. They agreed to install the super sports model Pacemaker, only recently on the market. In spite of having several years left on my old Pacemaker battery, it was not really meant for people with such an active life as mine. Replacement was a quick day surgery requiring only local anesthetic. They cut a slit in my chest, pulled out the old device, slipped in the new one and I was out in a couple of hours.

Now there would be no more heart problems - right? But it really never ends.

Travel the World

I married Brian, a long-time friend of Chris' and someone whom I had known for over twenty-five years. Our mutual interest in travel and seeing the world was the glue to an emerging affection that was developing. Brian was unconcerned with my heart history or the scars that remained and I had relegated it to the back of my mind. We moved to China in 2002 and then to the Middle Eastern country of The United Arab Emirates in 2003. We were living our dreams of seeing the world, as we used our new locations to see places we had barely dreamed about. It would be years before my heart health became an issue, and it started from somewhat unrelated issue. Following are two stories Brian wrote for a book about our world travels.

Hospital Holiday
July 2010

The summer of 2010 saw us heading into our final holiday as residents of the United Arab Emirates. We would be sorry to leave our home for the past seven-plus years in the desert city of Al Ain, but the work environment had become too much for either of us to tolerate.

I could have handled more if it hadn't been for Rochelle's predicament. For almost two years, Rochelle had been the reluctant manager of the department at our college with the most faculty and the most students. She was neither qualified for nor interested in doing the job of Chair of the Work Readiness Program. However, she did an excellent job of excelling in an unmanageable situation. Perhaps her success was because she didn't really want the job and would have liked nothing more than to be relieved of her onerous duties. The stress had taken its toll on her health, and we were looking forward to a summer of rest and relaxation before returning for the final stretch.

I had just received a very lucrative offer to move to Doha, and although it would be easy for Rochelle to find meaningful work there, the plan was to have her relax for a few months before seeking work. We still had to return to Al Ain after the summer for one last semester before my Doha contract commenced in January.

Our summer plan was to start with a few days in Atlanta to visit my older son and then travel to Calgary to see my younger son and Rochelle's daughter. Then, we would go to Chicago where my older son would travel for his marriage vow renewal, and I would also attend a writer's conference to hone my skills. Following that, we would spend a few more days in Atlanta before spending our final month relaxing on the beach in Thailand. We didn't know when we began our journey that we would experience major modifications to our well-thought-out plan.

Rochelle was exhausted on the flight to Atlanta, and we both were happy to arrive at my son's home where we could unwind and get a proper sleep. Proper sleep never happened. Rochelle's "hangover" from her tough workload didn't go away. She tossed and turned and required several pillows to prop her up in a comfortable enough position to nod off on occasion before awaking to more discomfort.

We did a bit of touring in Atlanta with my son, his wife, and their children, but Rochelle had a tough time keeping up whenever we had to walk. She was no more rested at the end of these few days than she was when we left the Middle East.

Upon arrival in Calgary, Rochelle and I, as often happened in the summer, were whisked off in different directions. My son was at the airport to greet me and take me to his home while Lori did the same, taking Rochelle to her home. This reduced our communication to daily phone calls. The one day when we did get together was to take my grandson to a movie, and Rochelle couldn't keep up on the walk through the mall to the theater and required several rest stops.

Back at her daughter's place, Rochelle's daughter became so concerned with her mother's appearance that she took Rochelle to the hospital emergency room.

The nurse took one look at Rochelle exclaiming, "Is she always this colour?" Rochelle was pushed to the front of the several-hour queue to a bed in the emergency ward. Medical staff performed immediate tests on Rochelle because of her artificial heart valve and related pacemaker. Blood tests revealed that Rochelle's hemoglobin count was a dangerous seventy-seven rather than the normal one hundred thirty. She appeared to be losing blood and was in congestive heart failure. Rochelle was immediately admitted to the hospital.

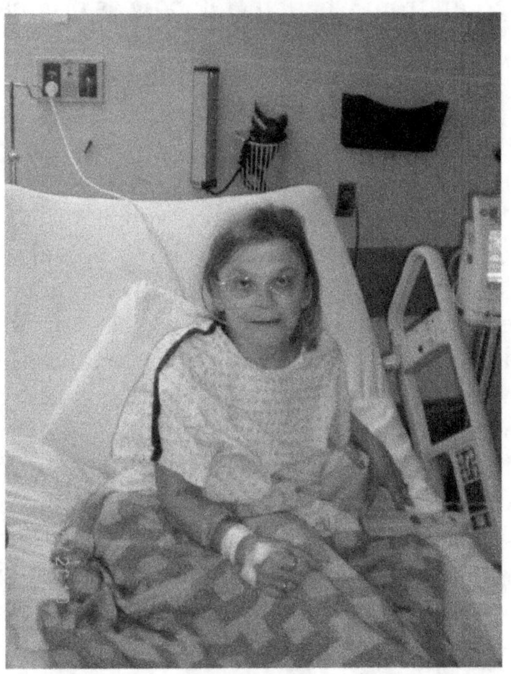

The beauty of the Canadian health-care system is that the first priority is the health of the patient rather than how the customer will pay, as is common in other jurisdictions. Money was never mentioned even though we could not produce an Alberta Health Care Insurance card. We showed them our medical insurance card from the UAE and nothing more was said.

Initial examination determined that Rochelle had blood in her stool that was originating either from her stomach or her bowels. She was bleeding to death and required transfusions to replace the lost blood. The transfusions brought her hemoglobin to an acceptable one hundred twenty. The next task was to ascertain from where the blood was originating.

The first procedure was an endoscopy to examine her stomach. When the doctors heard about our time in China, they suspected a bug that had been lying dormant for several years might be the culprit, causing bleeding ulcers. This theory proved negative, so the next step was a colonoscopy to see if the bleeding was originating from her bowels.

A colonoscopy requires complete eradication of everything from your bowels, so no food intake. In addition, Rochelle had to drink a chalky fluid to aid in the cleansing of her bowels—not a pleasant experience. Then she was given a drug to help her deal with the extreme discomfort of having a tube stuck up her rear. She was conscious during the procedure and experienced the discomfort in a haze, but she forgot most of it after its completion.

The procedure showed two polyps, one of which was four centimeters and had ruptured, causing the bleeding.

Normally, a doctor would remove the polyps during this procedure. However, Rochelle was taking blood thinners for her heart issues, and the doctor didn't want to risk further bleeding. At first, the doctor gave us the option of removing the polyps now or waiting until we returned to the UAE after they had brought her blood count to an acceptable level. We opted for the later procedure so we could salvage some of our holiday time.

However, continued excessive blood in Rochelle's stool removed the holiday option. The large polyp was still bleeding, and she would have bled to death before we finished our trip. So the doctor scheduled a second colonoscopy after they had sufficiently thickened her blood to avoid bleeding. This procedure was intended to allow the removal of the two polyps.

Now Rochelle had to go through a second uncomfortable round of cleansing her bowels and drinking the putrid brew provided by the pleasant, skilled, and helpful nurses. Another dose of the mind-numbing drug and she was taken away for the second probing of her bottom with the hopes of eliminating the source of her ailments.

Lori and I waited outside the operating room for Rochelle's emergence. Many other patients came and went, wheeled in and out of operating rooms with similar procedures but no sign of Rochelle. We began to worry and made nervous small talk to hide our fears.

Finally, after more than double the time of the routine procedure had elapsed, Rochelle was wheeled out in her bed. Although still groggy, she was visibly upset and very angry. The doctor told us that he had removed the smaller polyp but was unable to tackle the larger one due to its size and awkward location. He informed us that a specialist would have to remove the big polyp in a third procedure—thus Rochelle's anger at having to go through the detested routine again. In her delirium, she uttered unusually foul language and demanded an ambulance to take her away from all of this.

We had already used up nearly two weeks of our precious vacation time with no relaxation yet. Because of Rochelle's other issues, these normal procedures took much more time than would otherwise be expected because of having to thicken or thin out Rochelle's blood depending on what was being planned on any given day.

She was still receiving occasional transfusions to keep her blood count above the danger zone. In addition, she was getting several blood tests each day to monitor her blood thickness—thick for operating day and thin for recovery and eventual hospital discharge.

Next up, the third and, hopefully, last colonoscopy for the removal of the offending growth. A specialist from Toronto happened to be in town and was assigned the operation. This one went smoothly and quickly with the brash, self-assured, but obviously efficient doctor bragging to us about the procedure and how he had accomplished it. He even gave us a series of photographs of the polyp before and after and pointed out a "tattoo" he had placed at the site where the polyp used to be. It was only at this point that he asked about payment, as he was not part of the hospital billing system. He took a copy of our health insurance card from the UAE, and that was the last we heard about money.

Rochelle's bleeding problem was now history, and with some more transfusions her hemoglobin count was almost normal. Discharge from the hospital was now dependent on her blood thickness (INR), which had to be brought within an acceptable range. This magic number was reached within a couple of days, and we could now proceed with the rest of our holiday.

The Canadian health-care system was fast, courteous, and efficient. The hospital and the doctors billed our insurance company directly, so we didn't incur out-of-pocket expenses. The bill probably exceeded $50,000. Thank goodness we didn't go to a hospital in the United States.

Rochelle was discharged was Friday, July 2, and we had consumed almost three weeks of our summer holiday. We now planned to continue with our trip to Chicago and back to Atlanta. But we decided to cancel Thailand to allow Rochelle some recovery time back in Al Ain.

Rochelle was still very weak during our time in Chicago, where we had three events planned—Tony's vow renewal, his son's baptism, and my writing conference. The whole time Rochelle struggled to keep going, but we were able to accomplish all that we planned and even attended a couple of live theater performances. We hopped the plane for Atlanta where we still had a few days of visiting before returning home.

While Rochelle was sitting and catching her breath after the long walk to our gate at Midway Airport in Chicago, we both noticed a large swelling in her ankles. This was a sure sign that she was retaining fluid and might well be back in congestive heart failure. After arriving in Atlanta at my son's place, I made the decision to catch the next available flight back home to have Rochelle's health issue dealt with immediately. I didn't want to risk being caught in the black hole of the American health-care system, where green is the only colour that matters.

I had no trouble cancelling our Thailand trip for a full refund, and for a small change fee, Delta Airlines put us on the next direct flight to Dubai. We got home to Al Ain late at night, and the next morning went direct to Rochelle's heart doctor at American Hospital in Dubai. "American" is just the name; it actually has no affiliation with the United States in any manner. It is a luxury, private hospital that was connected to our health insurer for billing purposes.

Rochelle's doctor, whom she had just visited a month earlier and had given her a clean bill of health, rushed Rochelle into the emergency unit for testing and eventual admission to the hospital for further treatment.

The UAE health-care system is patterned after the US model with private hospitals and insurance. They will not proceed on most treatments without knowing where there money will come from. The biggest difference from the US model is that they seldom deny a claim. The hospital wanted to charge my credit card with a deposit, after receiving approval from the insurance company. I knew from our insurance provider previously that approval was usually immediate, so any delay was from the health provider not taking the time to ask the insurer. I stood my ground until they finally called the insurance company and got the necessary approval. After that, we were given excellent treatment with no mention of money.

Rochelle's major symptoms were shortness of breath and swelling in the abdomen and on the legs.

The first stop was the ICU (intensive care unit). Her heart doctor wanted to have her monitored continuously while diagnosing and treating her condition. She spent a couple of days in ICU, where she received diuretics to deal with the obvious fluid retention and an increased dosage of her blood thinner. She never achieved the optimum level of blood thickness after her procedure in Calgary.

Further testing showed that her pacemaker was working fine, but her heart was not able to work hard enough to expel the fluids from her body. So, the doctor increased her heart rate on the pacemaker from sixty beats per minute to seventy beats per minute for the lower limit. That combined with the diuretic seemed to fix the fluid-retention problem. The only thing that concerned me about the increased heart rate was that the suggestion came from me. I had asked the doctor if that would help, and he did it. Why didn't he figure it out first?

As a precaution, Rochelle was fully examined for complications from her colon procedures in Calgary in addition to a check of her gall bladder. Everything else was fine.

She was then transferred to a regular ward unit (more about those facilities below) for a couple of days of monitoring. Her breathing returned to normal, and the fluid seemed to be completely gone. At that point she was just suffering from extreme fatigue and weakness from the ordeal of the past two months. Rochelle's tiny frame had lost over 15 percent of its mass and she was skin and bones. As some might say, she was "a pirates' dream—a sunken chest."

American Hospital in Dubai

This is a story in itself, especially contrasted with the hospital in Canada. Rochelle's stay and treatment was all covered by our insurance, but I would have to pay for any nights I stayed and any meals I consumed. This seemed fair.

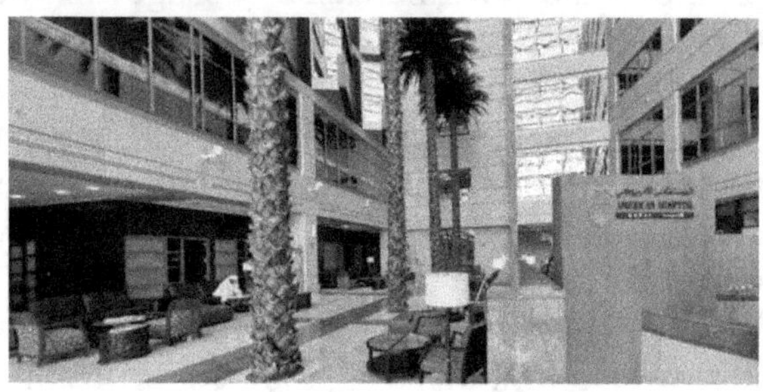

Emergency ward

Rochelle received immediate and continuous care when admitted to the emergency ward. She had her own room, and for the longest time, she was the only patient in emergency. There was one doctor, an assistant or intern, a couple of nurses, some porters, and an administrator all dealing with her issues. Once they received the approval from our insurance carrier, they moved her to the ICU.

ICU (intensive care unit)

Once again, Rochelle had her own room with her own toilet for her two night stay. Not luxury accommodations but the room was better than many hotels I have stayed in. There was no extra bed, but there was a fancy recliner that I could rest and even sleep in. I spent one night there. The other night, I had to return to Al Ain to attend to personal affairs. The nurses don't work like they do in Canada, but then I don't think they have the capacity to do some of the intense work that the Canadian nurses have to do. Each nurse was assigned two rooms, which means two patients. They took care of regular monitoring and administration of medication, but other than that they were more like maids, fetching whatever you needed. They wouldn't let you do anything for yourself, including retrieving ice.

Regular ward

I wouldn't put it in the category of a five-star hotel, but it was far superior to many three- and four-star hotels I have stayed in and was considerably more comfortable than the acceptable ICU. Rochelle had a regular hospital bed, but the rest of the room was more like a hotel. There was a large built-in sofa that I could use for sleeping. There was a built-in desk with Internet access, but I had to provide my own computer. We had a private toilet with shower and a large picture window overlooking a beautiful courtyard. The nurses were not overworked. We hardly ever saw a nurse, but they were available if you needed them—mainly for fetching pillows, blankets, etc. Rochelle was hooked up to a mobile monitoring device, so her readings were transmitted wirelessly and continuously. Other than daily blood work and administration of pills and injections, the nurses didn't have to do much. They certainly didn't have the patient load that a Canadian nurse would have, neither did it seem that they had the same competence, nice but dumb. Many of them spent their days playing games on the computers at their desks. Again, we were both served meals from the cafeteria after putting in our daily requests.

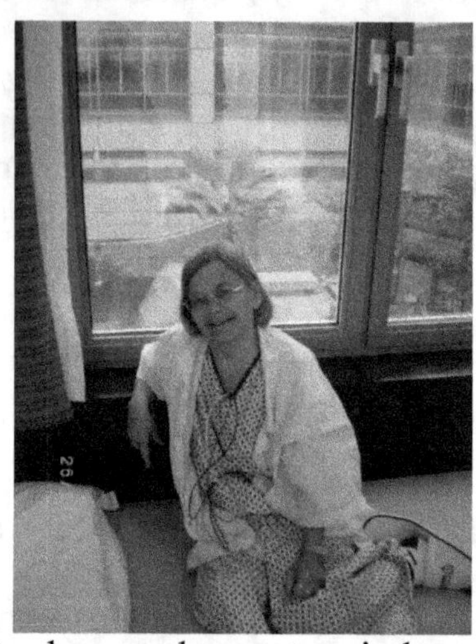

I don't know how to judge hospital equipment, but it appeared that the hospital had some of the best equipment that money could buy. It was always available, and it didn't seem to get much usage. Compare this to the hospital in Calgary that was always bustling. The Arab doctors seem to be very competent, helpful, and friendly. Although of Arabic background, they were all American trained and certified, with extensive experience in the United States.

The biggest problem for me was the daily drive when I didn't stay the night. It's a long drive from Al Ain to Dubai, and the road was under major construction.

Rochelle was finally discharged July 26, leaving only a couple of weeks of holiday time to recover before our final semester in Al Ain. The insurance covered the treatment and the bill for my extras amounted to the equivalent of about twenty-five Canadian dollars.

Here is Rochelle's summary of the ordeal, written immediately after her discharge:

Hello!
Yes, I'm still here!

As you all know last year was a stressful year for me. Once I took on the job as chair of the department (which I didn't want to do), I was determined to make a difference. I did get a lot accomplished and got lots of praise.

But by the end of the year, I was totally exhausted...I could hardly wait to get to Lori's and just relax. Brian would stay with Cam's (his younger son's) family while Lori and I would take it easy.

When I got to Lori's, she took one look at me and said I looked awful. I told her I just needed a few days and I would be fine.

Well, after a few days, I still had no energy, I wasn't sleeping, and I wasn't eating. Lori said, "We are going to emergency to get things checked out."

In emergency, they found my red blood cell (hemoglobin) count was seventy-seven (normal is over one hundred twenty) and I had fluid on my lungs. The reason my blood count was so low was that I was hemorrhaging somewhere inside. They admitted me and it was decided they would look at my stomach (bleeding ulcer) and my colon (colonoscopy). I was given three pints of blood to perk me up and a strong diuretic to get rid of the fluid.

The endoscope (look at the stomach) found no trace of an ulcer. However, the colonoscopy uncovered two polyps, but because I am on blood thinner they were afraid to remove them until my blood was thicker.

The next day I underwent a second colonoscopy. Brian and Lori waited outside, as they had during the first one, I was not a happy camper. After ninety minutes, I was wheeled out, and we were told they only removed one of the polyps. The other was too difficult to remove in its current location, and they booked a third colonoscopy with a specialist for the next day.

Brian and Lori had their hands full, as I was extremely angry and was letting any doctor or nurse around know it.

The next day, the specialist was able to remove the large polyp, but as you can imagine I was totally exhausted. On top of already being run down, I had just gone through three colonoscopies and one endoscopy.

They kept me in the hospital to get my blood thin again and check fluid retention. Finally, after ten days they let me out.

But, *as you can imagine I was in not good shape. They had found why my red blood count was down, and why I was exhausted. They had fixed that but, I still had no energy, no stamina.*

And it was decision time;

We were to leave for Chicago and Brian's grandson's baptism and as well as a vow renewal for Tony and Lisa. Do I stay and rest at Lori's and have my heart checked to make sure it is OK. or do I go back home alone to Dubai and have my heart doctor check out things, or *do I go on to Chicago and take it easy until we get back to Dubai?*

Well, I decided to go on. I told Lori, Rob, and Brian that it was my choice. Maybe not the smartest choice but my choice. It was what I wanted to do.

So we went on to the family. I was not at my best and took things slow.

When we got back to the UAE, we immediately went to my heart doctor. He, of course, put me in the hospital in Dubai straight away and checked out my heart and pacemaker. They did some adjustment to the pacemaker to make it work harder, and I am going to be on diuretic pills for a while.

Now, it seems all I need is time to regain my strength. Hopefully, within a month I will have my energy back and feel like my old self.

Hamad Heart Hospital

Another Middle Eastern country and another Middle Eastern hospital
September 2011
A hair-raising story in three parts:

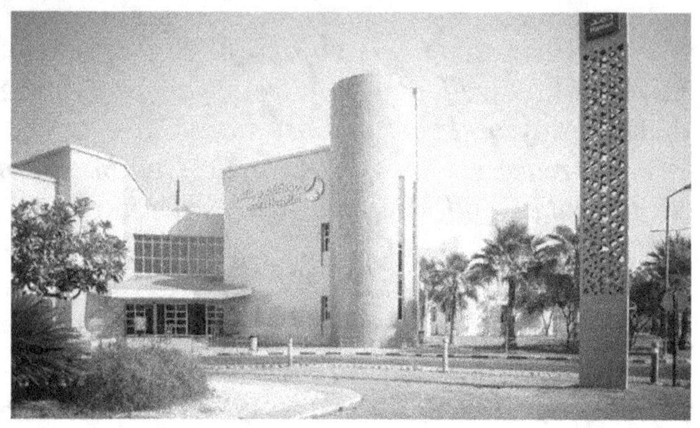

Part 1—background and admission

We moved to Doha in January 2011, and by spring Rochelle had located the only pacemaker clinic in the city at Hamad Hospital, a government-run institution among a plethora of private hospitals all within walking distance of one another.

At her June appointment, Doctor Saeed at the pacemaker clinic reported that there was still eighteen to thirty months left on her current pacemaker, which had been installed in Calgary about ten years earlier; it had served her well. He said, however, that she should come back right after our summer vacation to have it checked again, and he would keep monitoring it every month thereafter. Her first trip back in September showed a reading of "ERI," or elective replacement indicated. This message had replaced the normal message giving the number of months remaining in the life of the device. ERI is one step before the message "EOL," meaning end of life. I'm not sure if that means end of the life of the unit or the end of the patient's life. Regardless, Doctor Saeed said it was time to get a new unit—and soon.

What followed was a series of appointments and tests at the pacemaker clinic and the Hamad cardiology unit. Up to this time, I had not been directly involved as Rochelle's appointments were always during my working hours. Rochelle always came back from these appointments frustrated, confused, and in a tizzy. It sounded like disorganized chaos at the hospital. So, I tried to get her to schedule appointments when I could come along and get the information first-hand.

My first visit showed my some of the reasons for Rochelle's state of mind. First of all, Rochelle went into full panic mode even before reaching the hospital. Her normal calm, mature demeanour disappeared, and she became a blithering fool, unable to form full sentences and communicate a coherent message. The other reason I found out was that the hospital (and hospitals in general in Doha) are staffed with very nice and polite Middle Easterners and Asians who would have trouble understanding how to perform the duties of a Walmart greeter, let alone how to run a hospital. This definitely applied to all administrators, and for the most part the well-intentioned nursing staff. We did find a reasonable level of competence with the actual medical staff, especially the doctors.

We were greeted by these "nice" people who

immediately asked to see Rochelle's appointment card. This would be the start of setting Rochelle off because she was never given an appointment card. Doctor Saeed always had her phone his mobile as soon as she arrived at the clinic and he or someone would come and fetch her. It seemed like the medial staff didn't really want to rely on the administration, so they always had a "back-door" way of doing things.

After a series of fits and false starts, cancelled appointments, and other emergencies by the doctors, she was given an admission date—Tuesday, October 4. We arranged to go together right after work and get her admitted to the brand new Hamad Heart Hospital, a separate facility from the main hospital. So new, in fact, that the pacemaker clinic had not yet relocated.

As we entered the lobby, we were greeted by a well-dressed gentleman in a dark suit who welcomed us to the hospital and asked how he could help. I told him that my wife was being admitted for a pacemaker replacement. He asked for our admitting card, which, of course, we did not have. He then took us to a Qatari gentleman, dressed in his white thobe, who was the head of admitting. While I was dealing with these two gentlemen, Rochelle got on her mobile phone to Doctor Saeed. The whole lobby reeked of confusion and chaos. I was trying to explain to these two administrators that we were not issued an admitting card and that we always just called the doctor. Then Doctor Kassim, one of the heart doctors showed up. He exchanged a few heated words with the administrators in Arabic, and the only word I picked up was "emergency." Again, it was clear that Rochelle's doctors had their own plan for admission that didn't involve the front door.

Doctor Kassim whisked us away to the emergency ward where Rochelle was beset upon by at least a half a dozen nurses, who were all referred to as "sister." My immediate thoughts were that Larry, Curly, and Moe had a bunch of daughters and they all ended up as "sisters" at the Hamad Heart Hospital. These Asian (Filipina and Indian) ladies were tripping over each other to deal with Rochelle's "emergency."

They stripped Rochelle down, slipped a gown on her, put her in an emergency bed, strapped her up to every imaginable wire and gadget, and began firing questions at her. "How do you feel? Do you have any pain? Is your chest tight?" They started filling out forms and each nurse took a turn asking the same questions over and over again in broken English. Each of them wrote the answers on their form, but no one ever seemed to read the previous reports because this became a standard procedure for the rest of Rochelle's time in the hospital. She was repeatedly asked the same questions: "How long have you had this pacemaker? Do you feel dizzy? Are you on medication?"

Rochelle was the only patient in the emergency ward and had the full attention of every one of the plentiful staff who seemed to be just waiting for some emergency to beset them. Doctor Kassim had disappeared, and we were now left to the mercy of the daughters of Larry, Curly, and Moe. Before he disappeared, the doctor had assured us that Rochelle was scheduled for 8:00 a.m. the next morning to have her pacemaker replaced.

The emergency room doctor showed up and began to ask all the same questions that had been written on all the previous forms that he had never read. We were told that Rochelle would be sent to her room shortly because they had a quality standard of no more than a one-hour stay in the emergency ward.

The daughters of the Stooges then abandoned us to visit and giggle around the nursing station desks with a large dark-skinned gentleman in hospital garb, who resembled a character from a gangster movie. Other than the occasional visit from one of the mauve clad sisters, we were left alone to wait and wait. The one-hour quality standard had been exceeded considerably. I went to ask one of the nurses who was at the desk, and she said that the doctor had to sign the admission form.

I asked, "When would that be?"

She replied, "We don't know. We can't find him right now. He must be busy."

After another fifteen minutes, I asked the "gangster" guy when we would be going to a room, and he got on the phone right away. After about two and a half hours in the emergency, we were finally on our way to the wards to see more daughters of the Stooges in action. The next part of the story comes from the horse's mouth—the patient herself.

Part 2—the operation
In the words of the patient

Doctor Kassim, who admitted me and who has been involved since early on in the planning, came to see me on Tuesday evening to check on how I was doing and to give me the plan for the next morning—operation day. He assured me that I was going in at 8:00 a.m. the next morning. He also promised that he would come and see me the morning prior to the operation, telling the nurse to make sure I was ready to go for 8:00 a.m. He and Doctor Saeed (the pacemaker tech, maybe not even a doctor) were the only ones to instill any confidence that my operation could be successfully performed here.

True to his word, Doctor Kassim showed up at 7:00 a.m. Wednesday morning to tell me that everything was set for 8:00 a.m. and to re-inform the nurse to have me in the operating room at 8:00 a.m. Shortly before 8:00 a.m., I saw an orderly bring the transport bed and park it outside my room. Then I waited and waited. Finally, at 8:45 a.m. my nurse came in and started to get me ready to go to the operating room and wheeled me down in time for a 9:00 a.m. start.

I was wheeled into a little "holding" room where I was told to wait. Based on my experience to date, I wasn't confident that anyone would even remember where they left me.

As I lay there, I heard Doctor Kassim start shouting at my nurse, "I told you 8:00 a.m. I put it on the chart, 8:00 a.m. I reminded you this morning that it was 8:00 a.m. Look at the time. It's now 9:00 a.m. We are an hour behind, and we have two more procedures after this one. We almost had to cancel." He continued to berate and chastise the negligent nurse for several minutes, and I don't know to what end. The damage had already been done, and it was time to get to work. I was in fear that my procedure would be cancelled, and I didn't want to have to go through this chaos again.

Temped to jump out of bed and bolt for the door, I shouted out, "Hello. I'm in here. Are we ready to start soon?" After about ten minutes, they moved me into the operating room—over an hour behind schedule.

I was surrounded by five nurses, all busy doing nothing productive and arguing about whose job was what. Doctor Kassim and Doctor Saeed were both present in addition to a heart surgeon plus a couple other assorted males, bringing my entourage to about ten people.

Everyone seemed to have a task: setting up monitors or IVs, setting up the operating table, and prepping me for the upcoming procedure. It was chaos with lots of fussing and arguing. Next, the nurses started to fiddle with my clothes and bedding and then one of them shouted, "OK, all the men out, now." One of the few times the nurses had any ability to tell the doctors what to do. The males all dutifully exited the room while the females, all Indian nurses, continued to fuss over my "appearance." It was their job to make sure that I was appropriately covered in all the right places, so none of the men could get corrupted by a glimpse of any of my personal parts. When all the modesty coverings were in place, the men were summoned back to the operating room. Thank goodness there had been no emergency in the meantime; these nurses were obviously trained at the "Larry, Curly, and Moe Academy of Nursing." They instilled no confidence whatsoever.

Upon re-entry to the operating room, Doctor Saeed looked at the scene and blew a gasket.

"I told you her pacemaker is on her right-hand side. You have set up the whole procedure on her left. Get that fixed and now." The nurses hopped at the order and moved all the paraphernalia to the other side of the operating table. Again, the door looked very tempting—maybe I could catch a 10:00 a.m. plane to Sanityville. Doctor Saeed could see I was agitated and restless. Big deal; it's only my life at stake. He tried to calm me and said that everything was under control.

Now Doctor Kassim took charge of the task of hooking me up to a temporary external pacemaker. Being 100 percent reliant on the pacemaker in my chest, I couldn't afford to be without an electrical impulse to my heart for even one minute. I knew they talked about a temporary pacemaker, but I wasn't really clear on how they would do this. Nothing so far resembled my previous procedures years ago in Canada.

Doctor Kassim took a scalpel and sliced into my inner right thigh. I could see on the monitor as he pushed a wire through my vein to my heart.

"A little to the left. No, right. OK. Looks good," someone barked as Doctor Kassim pushed.

"Now, let's see if this works," Doctor Kassim proclaimed. I wished he would keep his commentary to himself. What if it didn't work? What was the back-up plan then? Then cheers erupted as he flipped the switch and the beeper started to go, and the waves appeared on the screen. This was supposed to be a standard procedure, not a shuttle launch. Being hooked to the machine as I was now removed any further temptation to run for the door, which still looked appealing given the gong show I was experiencing. I had flashbacks to my ordeals in Cyprus, London, and Karachi and thought how this made those experiences pale by comparison. I was in fear for my life as Doctor Kassim gave the signal to the heart doctor to disconnect my current pacemaker that had kept me alive for the past ten years. Again, more faint cheers from the crowd as I had survived another milestone, still alive.

The heart doctor, who never did reveal his identity probably for security reasons in case I expired, then started to cut into my chest to start the process of removing the old unit.

"Scalpel," he demanded of the nearest nurse. "Scissors," he continued. "Screwdriver." Wait! Did he say screwdriver? What the hell does he need with a screwdriver? Are a tire iron and hammer next?

He dug and gouged for what seemed like an hour. I was pushed and pulled in every direction as he tried to extract this piece of metal that had actually become a part of my body. I don't ride roller coasters, but I'm sure this was a worse ride. Then it popped out and he held up the bloody, tissue encrusted plate and showed it to me.

"See, this is what was inside you," he announced with a certain degree of pride.

I don't know why, but I instinctively replied, "Can I keep it?"

"Sure," he said as he passed the contraption to a nurse to clean it up for me.

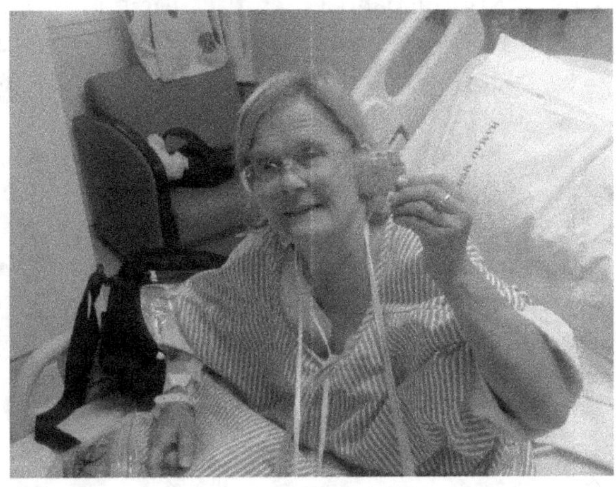

Now for the new, modern smaller model to take the place of the old clunker. Doctor Heart again started to prod and push, exclaiming that he couldn't make it fit. Why can't these guys keep their mouths shut when they are doing this?

"Maybe if you turn it this way," said one of the extra doctors.

"Put it in the other way," offered another. More confidence-building commentary making me wish that I had just let the old one run its course.

But eventually he got it in and turned on, and they disconnected the temporary external machine, and I was still breathing. The worst was now over.

"Pass me the glue," he continued and proceeded to "glue" my incision shut, fanning it dry with a piece of paper.

They wheeled me into the "holding" room and said my nurse would come to get me. I've seen this movie before. I wasn't about to be left stranded and abandoned in some holding tank.

"My husband is waiting for me," I barked. "I need to get to my room now." I asserted my authority.

"She will be here in a minute," the attending nurse informed me.

"No," I insisted. "Call her now. I can't wait here." Shortly, my nurse did show up and wheeled me back to my room where Brian had been pacing for four hours with no word about my ordeal. But it was over and now just the healing remained.

Part 3—the discharge—by Brian

Originally scheduled for Thursday, the day after the operation, Rochelle's discharge was delayed because we were waiting for her blood to reach the right level of thickness. She takes warfarin to thin her blood because of her artificial valve. Other than the occasional follow-up visit from the doctor, all she could do was wait until they said she was ready. That gave her lots of time to observe and be entertained by the comedy act that passed for hospital procedures. Fortunately, she had a private room, so she could close her door as needed. Much of the time she was hooked up to IV that pumped blood thinner into her system, thus restricting her freedom of movement.

The ward was full. Every room had someone in it, and there was an overabundance of nurses except when they were needed or wanted. The call buzzers were going constantly as were the phones at the nurses' stations. All of which went unanswered all the time. Doctors even complained to the nurses, "Don't you ever answer the phones?" Not when there is visiting to do or a coffee break or meal time. There were times when half a dozen of the "sisters" could be seen hanging around the nursing station while buzzers and phones were polluting with air with unnecessary sound. Other times, you could walk the length of the ward and never see a nurse. When they were around, they had a standard sct of answers for all questions that were designed to get the patients off their backs. Patients were such a nuisance.

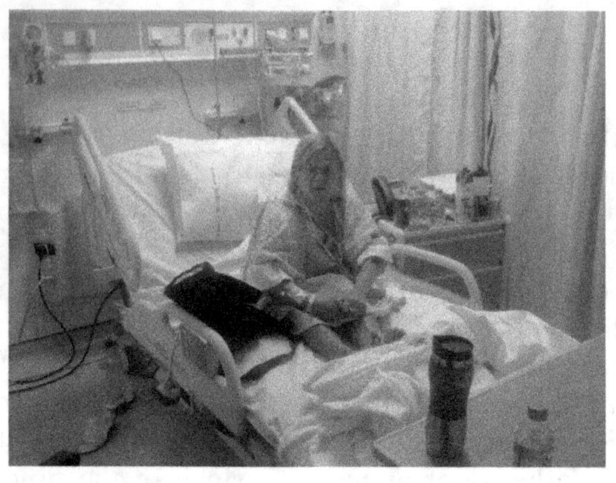

Friday morning, the doctor gave the word that Rochelle could go home; all was well. Now how long to get out of this den of comedy? Rochelle and I sat and waited for something to happen to let us know we could leave. Rochelle decided to get dressed to try to speed things up, but she needed to get all the contraptions removed from her body.

When she asked the nurse to do this, the nurse said, "Just a minute," and then disappeared faster than a Carrefour "may-I-help-you" worker (that's another Middle Eastern service story). Finally, all the prods and probes were removed, and we waited some more.

"What's the hold up now?"

"The doctor must sign the forms."

"Call the doctor."

"We don't know where he is."

The nurses have minimal training, low motivation, and absolutely no authority. They are constantly berated by their Arab patients and the superior doctors, so they are motivated to just stay out of the way and not be seen. They do this very well.

But they definitely don't want to overstep their bounds and get in trouble with anyone who might be their superior—which is actually everyone.

I saw this as an opportunity to speed things up and told the nurse, "We're leaving now. I'll give you my number, and you can call us when the doctor shows up." This announcement horrified the nurse, who got on the phone right away and tracked down the doctor. She didn't want to be responsible for an escaped patient.

Finally, we were on our way home for healing and recovery. We tried to keep ourselves healthy and fit for the rest of our time in Doha. This was not the place you wanted to be sick and in hospital.

First Signs
March 2017 Hospital Trip

My heart seems to get the seven-year itch. I had just turned seventy years old and we had finished couple of warm weather holidays to escape the harsh Canadian winter. Brian and I retired to Calgary in 2014 and were enjoying our freedom and love of travel with trips to a variety of Asian countries, some Central American countries, as well as destinations in the Untied States. In March, 2017 we had just stepped of the plane in Calgary from an enjoyable trip to Arizona, when I felt a pain in my shoulder and shortness of breath, resulting in a slow shuffle through the airport to our taxi.

Our regular and reliable family doctor, Dr. Shaub, was unavailable, so I visited his substitute to find out what was happening with my health. He wasn't particularly helpful but sent me for an x-ray on my shoulder and scheduled an echo-cardiogram. After a week of no answers and no solutions and no improvement in my condition, Dr. Schaub, who had returned, recommended that we go to emergency at the Foothills Hospital, recognized as being THE heart hospital in Alberta.

After an all-nighter in emergency, where I was subjected to a series of tests and lots of waiting, I was admitted to the heart ward for further examination - there was something wrong with my heart. I left hospital after two weeks of testing and observation, but didn't really have any answers. I did have a dozen new medications to take four times each day.

I felt I left the hospital in worse shape than I entered. I even made an appointment with the Pacemaker clinic to verify that my Pacemaker was not at fault. The Pacemaker was working fine, but there was only two years left on its battery life.

A few weeks later, Dr. Schaub again suggested that we make another trip to emergency. After several hours of tests and doctor visits, I was none the wiser. I was sent home with a minor tweak in my medications and an invitation to attend the cardio-rehab program at the fitness centre near our home. I was feeling more like an invalid every day.

Am I Cured?
May 2017 Hospital Trip

My five-hundred meter walk to the gym for my cardio-program was as much of an effort as the workout itself. One day I had to stop and rest several times on the short walk to the gym. It was clear that I was retaining fluid, as my feet and ankles began to expand. Another trip to Dr. Schaub convinced him that more aggressive action was needed. He personally phoned the cardio ward at the Foothills Hospital and arranged for a direct admission, bypassing the normal emergency process. By that afternoon I was in a bed in unit 8-2 of the Foothills Hospital.

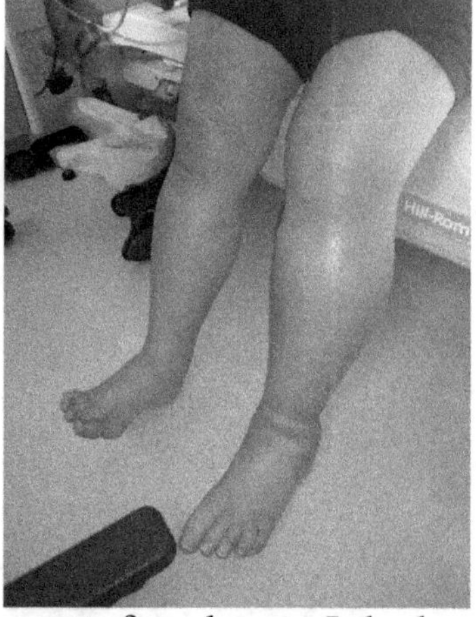

Over the next few hours I had continuous visits from members of the cardiology team and underwent several tests. Although there was no official diagnosis, the cardiologists determined that my body contained over eighteen liters of excess fluid. One look at my elephant legs was enough to confirm that fact, if not the quantity. My normal ninety-pound frame had given way to a near one hundred ten pound slow moving carcass. Cardiologists made minor tweaks to my medications, but the major treatment was aggressively attacking the fluid retention with a diuretic, administered through an intravenous feed. This plus an increase in my Pacemaker rate from sixty beats per minute to seventy beats per minute was sufficient to expel the excess fluid, and bring me close to my previous healthy self. The hospital stay was successful in attacking my symptoms, but the underlying cause was still a mystery - to me, anyway.

Dr. Kannani, my cardiologist whom I hadn't seen in two years, was on duty at the hospital during part of my hospital stay. I had daily visits from the cardiologist team and Dr. Kannani was there for some of those visits. He began filling me in on results of the multitude of tests I had been undergoing. My tricuspid valve was leaking. This might be partly due to the insertion of my Pacemaker lead which was installed through this valve to the interior of my heart to deliver the pulse that kept my heart beating. Dr. Kannani felt this lead may be the cause of the leak, and replacing the Pacemaker system with one or more leads on the outside of the heart, may alleviate the problem. Given that I only had two years left on my current Pacemaker this sounded like a timely option. He sent me for more tests.

The next day, Dr. Kannani came into my hospital room with a sombre look in his face, looked me in the eye and said, "I'm so sorry." I stood stunned, looking back at him with a confused feeling throughout my body. *"Sorry for what?"*, I though. He continued to explain that my tricuspid valve was not just leaking, but was actually gushing. This valve is supposed to keep blood from regurgitating back to the side of the heart that had just been expelled. Most of my blood was flowing back to the side of the heart it had just vacated. Medication could not correct this problem. Diuretics and other medications could help for a while, but eventually the heart would fail and my symptoms would return, impairing my quality of life – and ultimately ending my life.

I began to hyperventilate; my head began to spin and my legs turned to jelly. I could barely exude the words through my tears, "How long? Five years? Two years?"

Dr. Kannani's rapid exhale almost sounded like a sick laugh, which of course it was not. "Heaven's no. Not that long," he blurted without giving thought to the impact of his words. "I doubt that surgery is an option. It is very high risk, given your background, and I'm not sure any surgeon would risk it. However, I will ask a heart surgeon to stop by and talk to you." With another sincere, "I'm so sorry," he exited my room, leaving me and Brian, who had been at my side during the conversation, with our mouths gaping. In continued to hyperventilate through the tears that were spouting from my eyes.

Not long after, heart surgeon Dr. Kidd stopped by for a visit and get a sense of my condition and outlook. I had regained some of my composure so I could talk sensibly to him. and demonstrate my desire for a long life. He said he would take a look at my case and decide if he would consider doing my heart surgery.

A group of heart surgeons and related medical staff met twice weekly to review cases and make recommendations. This committee, including Dr. Kidd, reviewed my situation at their next meeting and thought it worthy of further consideration. They sent me for more tests. After the tests, the committee revisited my case and one of the cardiologists came to tell me that the committee had rejected my case as being too risky. Devastated may be too strong a word, but I was more than a little disappointed to hear this news. They assessed the risk of failure (chance of dying on the operating table) as thirty percent - way above what they would consider an acceptable risk.

Dr. Kidd came into my room and sat down for a chat. I thought he was going to just confirm, in a gentle way, what I had just heard from the previous doctor. To my surprise, he did just the opposite. He said the committee assessed the risk at 30%, but having met and talked with me, which the others had not done, he could reduce the risk to below 10% - still high but acceptable. No surgeon wants to have a dead patient on their record. He told me to think about it and make an appointment to see him in his office after I was discharged from hospital and we could discuss the options and make a decision.

My two week stay in hospital had returned me to at least as healthy as I was before my heart issues had surfaced earlier in the year and I was discharged with another boatload of medications. My stay in hospital was made much easier with the daily help and support of Brian, Lori and Lori's partner, Grant.

I was able to return to the cardio program at the gym and begin to live a normal life again. All was well.

The Decision – Summer 2017

I left the hospital at the end of May 2017 feeling fifteen years younger. My weight was the lowest it had ever been in my adult life. I had almost endless stamina. I finished my twelve-week cardio program at the gym with almost no effort.   I continued my daily workouts at our gym which were minimum forty-five minutes long and sometimes well over an hour. After Brian and I finished at the gym, we would walk along the river and go sit for a coffee before walking home. Our routine trips to our family doctor were a chance to show off my stamina - I walked the five-kilometer round trip to the downtown clinic. In my mind, and according to how my body was responding, I was cured and healthy. I could live like this - forever.

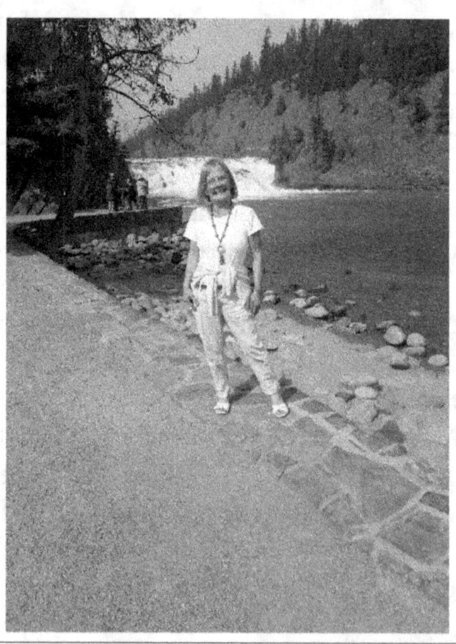

I made my visit to Dr. Kidd for the discussion about surgery. He was still more than willing to do the surgery and felt that it would provide me with long term benefits. But the decision was mine to make. I decided I wanted to go without surgery for as long as possible. My Pacemaker would have to be replaced in two years so that might be a good time to revisit the surgery decision. With Dr. Kidd's blessings, I decided to defer the surgery decision until I started showing signs of heart failure or until the Pacemaker needed replacing. Dr. Kidd sent me for some more tests to establish a baseline for future reference.

At a follow up visit to the Pacemaker clinic, Dr. Gillis recommended that my one-lead Pacemaker be replaced with a multi-lead model. Although this decision could be deferred until my current Pacemaker needed replacing in two years, she recommended an earlier replacement. This would not require surgery, but rather a less invasive procedure through the veins. The risk in this procedure was that the old lead (twenty years embedded in my heart) needed to be removed. Although this was supposed to be routine, they would keep a team of heart surgeons handy in case they had to open my chest if anything went wrong. Something seemed redundant about this option, as that would solve the Pacemaker problem, but I still might need further surgery to repair or replace my failing valve. Why not do both procedures at once? I decided to defer this decision until at least the fall.

My follow up appointment with Dr. Kannani changed everything. Recent tests showed that my tricuspid valve was leaking as bad as ever. Dr.

Kannani insisted that he had told me this when he first reviewed my file nearly three years prior. I don't doubt his word, but I also don't recall hearing anything about my dysfunctional valve until my last hospital visit. Dr. Kannani would not push for or against surgery, but he was quite emphatic that symptoms of heart failure (fluid retention, shortness of breath, chest pains) would return sooner rather than later. My two-year time-frame was unreasonable in his estimate. He even guessed that it might be only weeks or months for my heart to show signs of failure. A person can only live with a failing heart for so long, so his implication was that without surgery my life would be quite short. He suggested I have another chat with the surgeon, Dr. Kidd and if I decided on surgery, it would likely take place soon. This news forced me to rethink my earlier decision to defer surgery.

I met again with Dr. Kidd and told him that I had decided to go ahead with the surgery. Brian and Lori attended that meeting so they could hear his answers first hand and ask any questions they had. Dr. Kidd was surprised with my reversal and wanted to make sure I was making the decision for the right reasons. In the end, he agreed that it was better to do the operation now while I was healthy rather than wait until my heart failed. The surgery itself would be just as successful either way, but my chances of a good recovery and a healthy life would improve. He scheduled the surgery right on the spot, for only a matter of weeks away. He would contact the Pacemaker clinic to arrange to have the Pacemaker procedure done at the same time to avoid double procedures.

All was set, but I was scared. Was this the right choice? Dr. Kidd sounded confident, but didn't sugar coat the risks. There was still a chance that I wouldn't survive the operation and that if I did, it would be a tough recovery. I told him if he got me off the operating table, I would do the rest.

As the surgery date approached, blood tests showed that my hemoglobin level was low. This would increase the risks associated with the surgery, so Dr. Kidd deferred the surgery date by one month in order for me to go through a series of blood treatments to increase my blood count. As I have been on blood thinner for twenty years, I cannot have a medical procedure that might result in massive blood loss. So, I had to enter hospital early to make a transition from blood thinner to a different anti-coagulant. I entered hospital on December 3, 2017 to begin that process and get ready for surgery on December 5. No turning back now.

Day "O"

Upon admission to the cardio surgery ward, my nurse took Brian and me on a tour of the facilities and gave us the generic schedule of what to expect. I was admitted on the Sunday and my surgery was scheduled for Tuesday at 1:00pm. First, he showed us the family room - or surgery waiting room. Family of those undergoing surgery were invited to use that room, which had a phone to connect you to the Intensive Care Unit. The normal process was that once a patient entered surgery it was about a three-and-a-half-hour procedure. Family would wait in the waiting room as the surgery time was nearing an end and they would receive a call about thirty minutes prior to the end of surgery. When the surgery was complete, the surgeon would come and talk to the family to give the details of the operation and the expected recovery process.

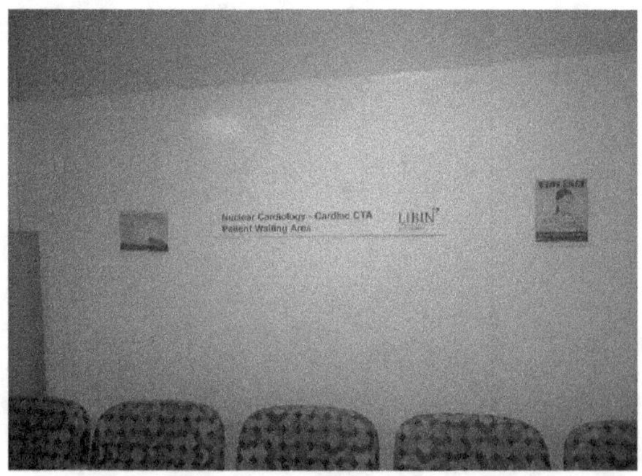

The family would then continue to wait in the room until they got a call from the ICU where the patient would be taken following surgery. The nurse showed us the door to the surgery unit and then the door to the ICU. Once the patient was settled into the ICU any family was permitted to come in and make a brief visit. After that, any visits to the ICU must be approved through phone contact and was limited to a maximum of two visitors.

The nurse then showed us the three post-ICU rooms where patients would go after their stay in ICU. After surgery, a patient went to the ICU for a day or two, then to post-ICU for two to three days, and finally a standard ward room for a couple of days before discharge. Many people were in and out of the hospital in a week. Most spent no more than ten days.

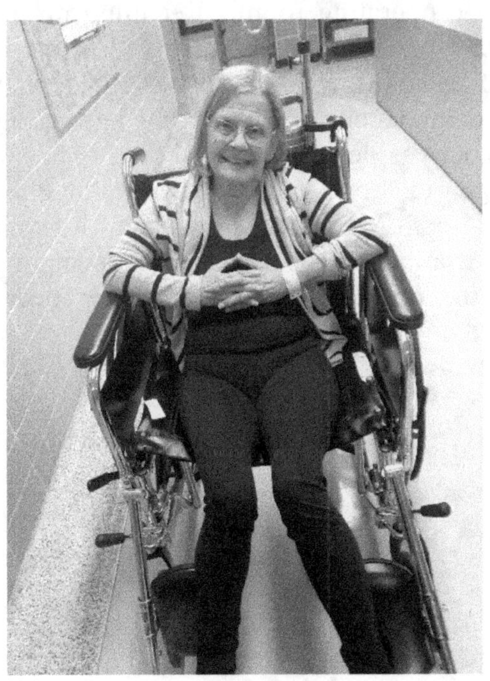

My non-standard situation was expected to be much longer. The length of my operation was harder to predict. The standard three to four hours would not apply. Originally, Dr. Kidd estimated an eight-hour operation, but later settled on a five-hour prediction. My ICU stay was expected to be three days, followed by about five days in post-ICU and up to two weeks in a regular ward. With entry to the hospital on December 3 and the operation on December 5, I did not expect to be home by Christmas and was prepared to spend New Year's in hospital - but that was OK, as long as I survived.

I surrendered my glasses and my hearing aids to Brian and crawled onto the stretcher. Brian walked beside my mobile bed, as the porter wheeled me towards the operating room. Recalling my previous operation, I made Brian promise to tell me, when I awoke (if I awoke), what day it was. My anxiety gave way to a calm, serene, almost giddy demeanour as the pre-op sedatives permeated my body. The overhead lights began to shiver and blur as my thoughts turned to relaxing on a Mediterranean beach. I gave a weak wave to Brian as my bed banged the swinging doors open to the operating room - I never heard them swing shut.

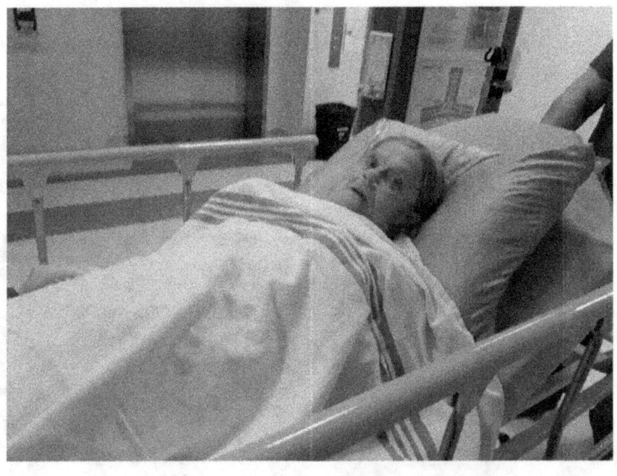

My next sensation was opening my blurry eyes and seeing people around my bed - nurses? Maybe family? Brian? Lori? Rob? I think I saw lips moving but absent my hearing aids and with my ears partly covered by some contraptions, I heard nothing. My blurred eyes shut and I disappeared into darkness.

I couldn't tell how much time had passed when my eyes next opened and I began to recognize people around me. Lips moved and I could hear fuzzy words entering my feeble ears. As my senses began to transmit information to my foggy brain, I began to interpret sounds, detect odours, and feel pain and discomfort. I couldn't lift my arm to remove the contraption from my mouth that was causing most of my discomfort. I drifted in and out of a wakeful state for a time frame that I had no ability to measure - Minutes? Hours? Days? I couldn't tell. Every time I felt a wakefulness, someone was beside my bed - usually Brian, Lori or Rob. They all showed concern mixed with optimism on their faces, and when I could hear and interpret the words, they were always encouraging and positive. The first words I actually remember was when Brian said to me, "It's Thursday, you went in Tuesday. You only lost two days." That was comforting, given my lost week the last time I was in this state.

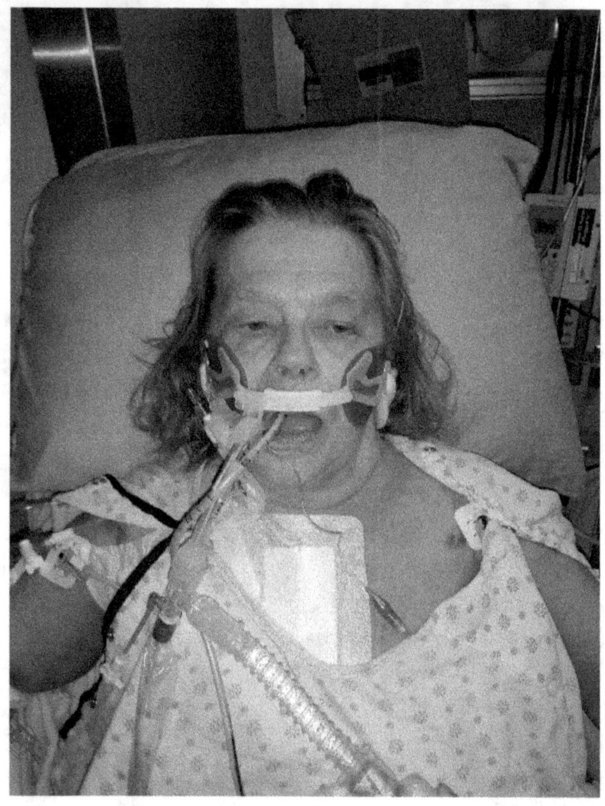

The Tube

I knew from Dr. Kidd and the anesthesiologist that once I was anesthetized they would begin hooking me to wires and tubes. One of the tubes I dreaded was the breathing tube down my throat. I recall from my previous operation waking to the tube in my mouth and throat, but it only lasted a day. Then I was rewarded with freezing ice chips in my mouth and to the back of my throat. I have loved ice ever since that operation.

I had told Dr. Kidd that all he had to do was get me off the operating table and I would do the rest – but this was going to be harder than I thought.

I felt the tube in my mouth and down my throat when I began to recover my senses. I wanted so badly to reach up and remove the invading contraption from my mouth, but there was always someone there to push my hand away and prevent my self-damaging behaviour. I could not hear what people were saying, but I could not respond. I hoped that I would have the tube removed within hours of my wakefulness, but that turned out to be a fanciful dream. The tube was destined to be part of my body for several days.

I had limited strength to lift my arms, and no ability to move any other part of my body. Not only was I acutely aware of my mouth tube, but I also became aware of the other multitude of other tubes and wires protruding from my body. Rob passed me a paper and a pen and I gained a method of communicating with those beside me. I could lift my arm enough to hold a pencil and write on a pad held by someone. Brian, Lori and Rob (until his departure to his home in Regina) took turns visiting me, sitting beside me while I napped. Each took their turns holding a notepad for me to tell them my thoughts and immediate needs. Most of my notes were of a maintenance nature: "I'm so tired"; "Pain killer soon?"; "Bum sore from sitting". However, others were more insightful or profound: "This is tougher than before"; "I am alive"; "Happy, thanks for everything". Sometimes it was just a complaint: "Shit"; "Boo"; "Tell the doctor I have the tube in for 6 days - no fair!!". I was occasionally even able to get off the odd funny: "How Sexy", in reference to having Brian wipe the drool from my mouth.

A series of notes to Brian described an incident during one of the evening shifts. It was based on facts that I could observe, but given my less than lucid state, it was intermixed with drug induced fantasy. A particularly difficult patient was wheeled into the ICU. He was likely high on drugs and caused no end of trouble for the nurses who were trying to keep him alive. Out of precaution, all other patients, including me, were hidden away behind their sliding curtains. I recall trying to part the curtains with my hands and feet to see what was going on, but that was likely part of the fantasy as I could not really move much. I also recall a figure dressed in black (the Grim Reaper?) looking in on me and telling me I would have to wait my turn - I was next. Entry to Hell? By morning it was all over and everything was back to normal.

The first couple of days of alertness, with the tube in my mouth, was torture. I kept getting indications that this might be the day the tube would come out, only to be disappointed when I ended the day with no apparent progress. After the first few days, I just accepted my fate and although I hated the tube, I tolerated it. The nurses and doctors said the tube was essential because of my weak lungs. The lungs tend to collapse during surgery and patients have the tube inserted to help them breath. My lungs were taking longer to recover than most. Respiratory technologists gave me regular and increasing tests to turn down the breathing assist from the machine that powered the tube. At first, a short test left me tired from trying to power my lungs on my own. Each test got a bit longer and I gradually responded better, but still not good enough to remove the tube. Nurses encouraged me to cough on occasion to strengthen the lungs and clear and mucus accumulation. Coughing was a strange experience with a tube inserted into my lungs. For one thing, the cough was almost silent. Also, when any phlegm was expelled, the nurse would pump another tube to pull it away.

On the morning of my eighth day in the Intensive Care Unit, I had a coughing spell. I began coughing and couldn't seem to stop. The next thing I knew, I couldn't breath - no air at all would enter my lungs. I had coughed the breathing tube almost out of my system, but it had lodged in my throat preventing it from pushing air into my lungs and preventing me from inhaling any air from the room - I was suffocating. By the time I was somewhat alert to my predicament, I had several doctors and nurses panicking over my head and face. Was it seconds or minutes? I couldn't tell, but when I became aware of my ears working, I heard one of the doctors say, "I've got it." I could see him holding the tube in his hand. The next sensation I experienced was a rush of air entering my lungs - I could breathe again. I could feel something covering my face - it was a large mask pumping refreshing air into my mouth and lungs. My tube was out - but for good? I could hear the doctors contemplating reinserting the tube, but were hesitant because this was a high-risk procedure. They decided to leave things as they were, for now, and see how I responded.

Barely thirty minutes after my "incident", Brian walked in, unaware of the events that had transpired, and gave a huge smile when he saw the mask on my face. Still unable to talk, I was able to smile back, beneath the plastic face mask and flip him two-thumbs-up.

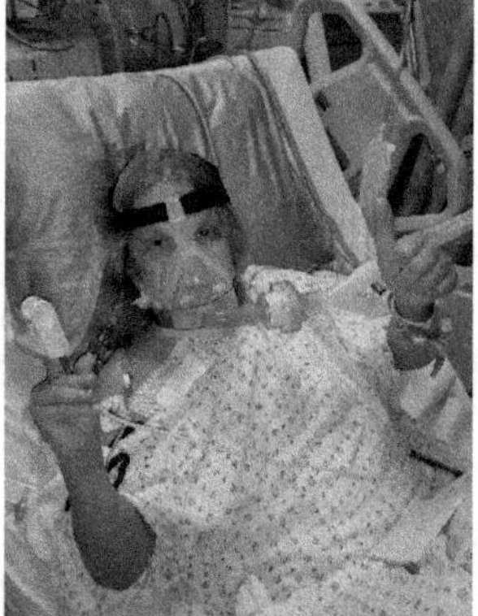

The nurse and a doctor gave Brian a brief synopsis of the morning events, conveying the gravity of the incident, exclaiming that they were very close to calling "Code Blue", meaning "patient in cardiac arrest". But for me, life was about to improve - the tube was gone. As the discharge report noted, "Patient self-extubated".

Post Tube ICU

The oxygen mask did not last very long. Because of my small size, including my face, respiratory technologists had a difficult time finding a mask to fit me. The big ones leaked everywhere and the small ones leaked in select spots, so their effectiveness was limited. In between attempts to find an appropriate mask, they put a standard tube to my nose, to at least get some oxygen into my lungs. They soon found out this to be adequate. My breathing stabilized and my oxygen levels were above acceptable levels. I could even go for periods of time with no supplemental oxygen. I was improving. My throat had some residual damage from having the tube into my lungs for so long - but this was expected to abate over time. I received my long-awaited reward of tiny ice chips tossed onto the back of my tongue. My voice didn't want to cooperate, but I was now able to communicate with a hoarse whisper, which exhausted me. The nurses were concerned with the condition of my throat relative to taking medications and nutrition. Part of my oxygen tube contraption included a tube to my stomach that allowed the nurses to administer food and medications. They decided to insert a small tube through my nose and into my stomach so they could get necessary substances into my system. Brian was not too keen on watching this process, so he took his regular break when they started the insertion process. Lori stayed on to observe the unsuccessful process. Right nostril - no luck. Left nostril - same result. My nose passage doesn't seem to conform to normal anatomy, so they abandoned the process. Nurses began administering my pills crushed up and in some pudding - it worked, I could swallow. With some careful attempts, the same happened with foods and fluids. I couldn't take much and it was quite an effort, but I could now take my meds and foods orally.

Late in the day of my "self-extubation", I observed the setting sun outside my window. The outgoing nurse conveyed to the incoming nurse the events of the day. With my raspy voice I told them that because of their efforts, I would see another sunset. Both nurse dribbled tears from their eyes saying they were just doing their job. I replied that in doing their job they had saved my life.

With my new ability to communicate, I was now able to piece together the forty-eight hours that did not form part of my memory. Brian in particular, filled me in on the drama that occurred from the time I entered the operating room, until my wakeful moments in the ICU.

After hearing all that had gone on during my lost forty-eight hours, and what I'd put my family through, I thought that both Dr. Kidd and I had gotten more than we bargained for.

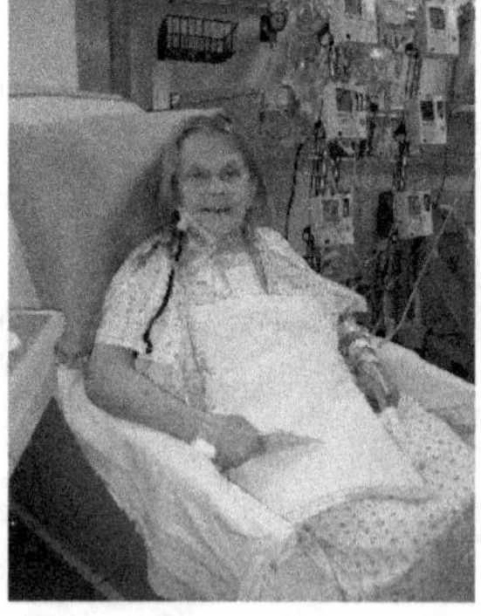

While You Were Sleeping

I entered the operating room at about 1:00 pm. With the expected five-and-a-half-hour operation I was to be out by about 6:30 pm. Brian, Lori, Grant, Rob and Annaliese gathered in the family room late in the afternoon to await the call. Other families also gathered in the family room to also await their calls. One by one each of the other families received their thirty-minute notice followed by a visit from their surgeon to fill them in on the details of the operation. Not long after they would receive the call that they could come to the ICU to see their loved one.

There was limited small talk as each of my loved ones processed the situation in their own way. As the time wore on, tension and stress filled the room which now had reduced numbers. At five and a half hours exactly - 6:30 pm, the phone rang in the family room asking for the relatives of Rochelle Bos. The operation was nearly over and Dr. Kidd would come out and talk with the family. Having watched other families go through the process, everyone became more concerned, as the thirty-minute time frame expired with no further word. Silence and sniffles filled the room. Lori had to take a couple of strolls to deal with her reddening eyes - Grant did his best to console her. Well after the thirty-minute deadline, the phone rang again for the Bos family, only to say that the operation was not yet done. Concern, bordering on dread, descended on the room as everyone waited on the fate of the high-risk operation. Lori's shaky strolls became more frequent. Then at 7:45 pm another phone call - it was over and Dr. Kidd would be out in thirty minutes.

Dr. Kidd surfaced at 8:15 pm - thirty minutes exactly since the last phone call. He looked tired and concerned, but not devastated. He set everyone's mind at partial ease by stating that I was OK. He then gave a brief synopsis of the operation. The key point was that there had been some post-operative bleeding that required immediate attention - thus the false alarm on the first call. They had packed my chest with material intended to help stem the bleeding and left my chest open until they felt the bleeding was under control - I had been moved to the ICU to await the next procedure. Dr. Kidd suggested a meeting with the family at 10:00 am the next morning to review the plan.

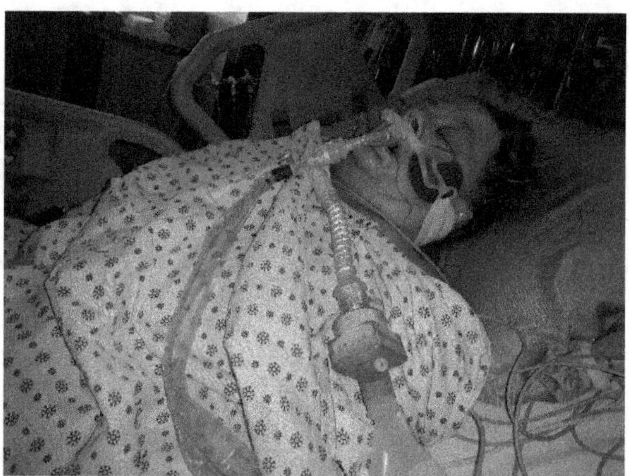

The five people closest to me (Anika was with a babysitter) were allowed to come in and see my immobile body lying on a bed with tubes and wires almost obliterating the presence of a human being. The ICU nurse was positive and optimistic, but made it clear that the next 48 hours was critical. After a short visit, less than the time one might view the guest of honour at a funeral. Everyone disbursed for the night for reassembly the next morning.

Dr. Kidd was right on time for the 10:00 am meeting. He relayed the events in the operating room the previous day. The fix of the tricuspid valve went mostly as expected with little incident. The removal of the twenty-year-old Pacemaker lead was not much of a problem.   But the installation of the new Pacemaker leads turned out to be more difficult than hoped. These leads were placed on the outside of the heart, rather than through a valve to the inside of the heart as with the previous system. Dr. Kidd installed four heart leads. The first one would not work at all, so he just left it there. The second one attached OK, but didn't really work. The next two worked fine, but the trauma to the heart and inside of the chest resulted in the bleeding that now left me in a comatose state with my chest open. One piece of good news he was able to relay was that the second lead that didn't work on installation was now working. There were now three functioning leads that helped my heart chambers to now beat in the proper order.   Prior to the operation, the chambers were not beating in sync, causing gradual damage to my heart.

The medical team planned to monitor my bleeding and see if they could get me back into the operating room later in the day to see if it was safe to close my chest. Everyone took a brief visit to see my immobile body before disbursing and awaiting my next procedure.

Closing the Chest

The medical team expected that I would return to the operating room at the end of the day (Wednesday December 6) to close my chest. It appeared that the bleeding in my chest was now under control, but as my next procedure was not urgent, I would re-enter the operating room after the regularly scheduled operations had been completed. Brian called the ICU on the morning after the operation to confirm that everything was OK and that I had a good night. He came to visit my comatose body and talked to the nurses and to Dr. Kidd, confirming the next step of closing the chest, which was expected to be a relatively short procedure. He then returned late in the afternoon and waited for me to go back in. I was still not in the operating room by early evening. In communication with the ICU, Brian found out that I had been pre-empted due to an emergency, and would likely not get back into the OR until the next morning. They suggest to Brian that he go home and check back in the morning, so he went home and crashed from all of the stress I was creating for those around me.

At 11:30 that night, Brian awoke to his ringing phone. Dr. Kidd called to let a groggy Brian know that my chest was now closed and everything worked out fine. I was back in ICU and would be allowed to wake up in the morning - Thursday morning, almost two days since first entering the operating room. By 10:00 am the next morning, Brian, Lori and Rob were beside my bed to see the first movement of my eyelids to indicate I was coming back to the real world.

Road to Recovery

I was still attached to a variety of hoses, tubes and wires, but the absence of the main tube down my throat allowed me to concentrate on getting myself better. Most days the nurses insisted I get out of bed and spend the day in an easy chair beside my bed. There I would sit, talking with Brian or Lori (Rob had returned to Regina) who took turns sitting beside me, or nodding off into a doze. In the evening the nurses moved me back to my bed, where I would sleep off and on, until the process repeated itself the next day.

The day after I accidentally (or was it?) forced the tube from my system, ten days since I entered the operating room, Brian walked beside me as the nurses presided over my graduation from the Intensive Care Unit to the post-ICU ward. I was still connected to a variety of appendages to my body, which followed me on a pole as the nurses pushed my chair to my new room. Although I initially had an oxygen tube sitting under my nostrils, it wasn't long before this became the first attachment to disappear. With limited help, usually from Brian or Lori, I could go for short walks with my pole and all of its wires and tubes. One by one, each of the attachments disappeared.

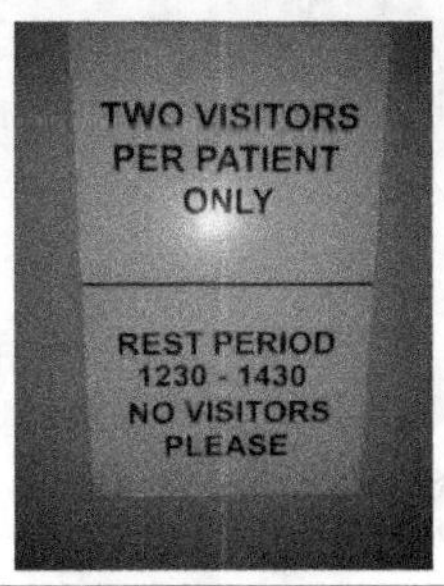

Every day I would anxiously watch and wait for Brian to arrive before 9:00 am and he would stay until after noon. He would catch me up on the latest political news, hockey scores, how he was sleeping and his workouts.

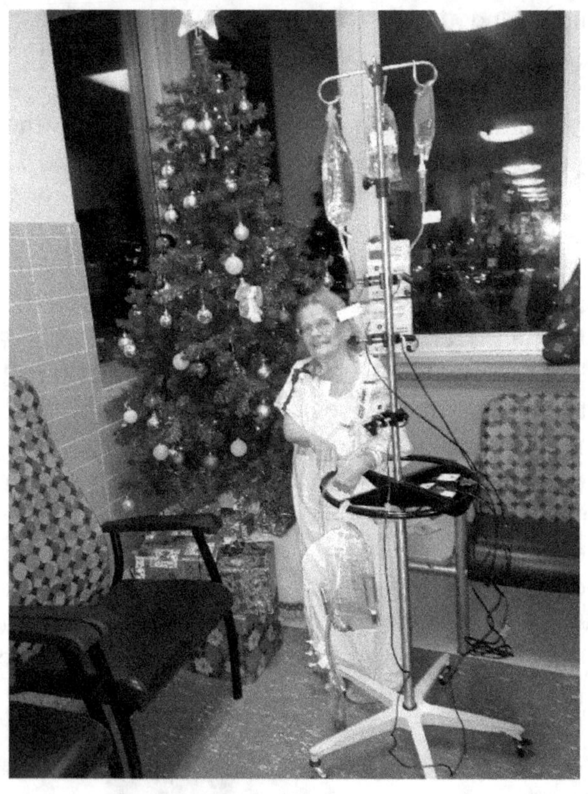

Then I would watch for Lori to arrive around 2:30 and she would stay until Brian arrived at 5:00. If I was not too tired Lori would come back in the evening. Sometimes Lori and I had deep discussions.

Had I made the right decision? Was she putting in enough time on her work?

They were my gophers – get me ice; where is my make-up bag; I want a cold face cloth; get my toothbrush; and so on. Sometimes I would just rest, close my eyes, and check to see that they were still sitting beside me or laying on the bed.

My focus was supposed to be on my own health and recovery, but my concern always turned to Brian and his health. Was he eating enough? Was he getting his exercise? He always shoved my concerns aside – but I pushed anyway. Lori, with Grant's prompting, prepared a huge dish of lasagna for Brian to eat, so I felt relieved to know he wouldn't starve.

Dr. Kidd came to visit a couple of times, usually just to say hi, but he did have one extended visit to debrief Brian and me on the entire process he had quarterbacked, and what we could expect moving forward. My tricuspid valve was still leaking and he explained in detail why. He was optimistic that although the tricuspid valve may never be perfect, it should improve and my post-op health should be better than my pre-op status. My new Pacemaker system was working fine, and with the alternating pulses coming from the three new leads, my heart should operate much better in the future.

Sleeping and getting a good night's rest was a nightmare, even with sleeping pills. Because of my breathing difficulties and fluid retention, I could not lay down flat, without panicking – sometimes a full panic attack. I slept sitting up, trying to get enough pillows to prop the bed into some sort of comfortable position – sometimes this seemed impossible.

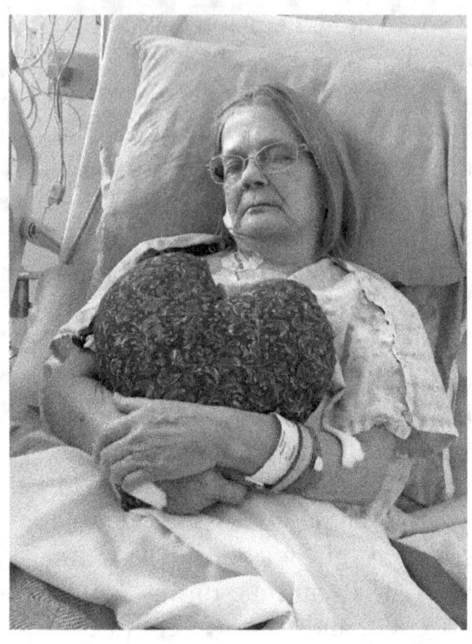

I had retained about fifteen liters of fluid since entering the hospital. This was quite common with heart surgery but was expected to gradually correct itself. My daily walks to the weigh scale confirmed that I was slowly losing the excess weight I had acquired during my post-op rehab. Soon I was down to just two attachments which pumped liquids into my body from my companion pole that was always at my side. These last two appendages disappeared by day seventeen of my ordeal, I was free of all attachments. I moved to a regular hospital room (ironically the same room I occupied on my admission) to await the all-clear for my eventual discharge. The diuretics and my leaky bowel forced me to wear Depends, so I had my son-in-law, Grant, make a trip to the hospital pharmacy to buy some feminine pads – imagine having to buy pads for your mother-in-law.

Most of my fluids were now gone but there was still a noticeable bulge to my ankles and feet. My nearly daily X-ray showed that there was still considerable fluid around my lungs, especially my left side. Although my aggressive diuretic intake would deal with this over time, the doctors felt that I would be better served with a quick drainage of the chest fluid. So, for about 36 hours I was outfitted with a tube inserted between my ribs on my back and into my chest to pull off the excess fluid. My laboured breathing improved almost instantly and when the tube was finally removed the doctors started talking about sending me home. Looking at my fat ankles and feet, I pushed back against an early departure. Given my experience earlier in the year, I was afraid of being sent home too early, only to have to be readmitted later.

The attendant doctor and associated nurse practitioner, assured me there was nothing more that could be done by keeping me in hospital and I would recover better at home than in hospital. They gave me the option of staying in hospital for an extra day or two, but did not advise it. I capitulated, and on December 24, the day before Christmas, nineteen days since my operation and twenty-one days since I entered the exact room in which I was currently residing, the attendant nurse processed my discharge papers, instructing me on my daily medication regime. Brian escorted me to the main entrance where I waited until he brought the car around.

Three weeks after the start of my ordeal, I was now free and on my way to a complete recovery. I knew I would be fine.

Appendix A - Time-line

1947 - Born with a heart murmur
1981 - Replace aortic valve with pig valve
1997 - Artificial valve - installed Pacemaker
1998 - Blew Pacemaker - in race
2000 - Blew Pacemaker - in Greece
2001 - Blew Pacemaker - in library
2001 - Replace Pacemaker
2010 - Congestive heart failure - bleeding polyps
2011 - Replace Pacemaker - in Doha, Qatar

2017
Problems:
March - Congestive heart failure
May - Congestive heart failure tricuspid valve failure
September - Decision to proceed with surgery

Surgery:
Dec 3 - Admission to Hospital
Dec 5 - Surgery for tricuspid valve and Pacemaker - internal bleeding, chest left open
Dec 6 - Bleeding stopped, chest closed
Dec 7 - Awoke from surgery
Dec 13 - Breathing tube removed - coughed out
Dec 14 - Moved to post-ICU ward
Dec 21 - Moved to regular ward
Dec 24 - Discharged from Hospital

Appendix B

Rochelle's notes – December 2017
The following are a partial listing of the multitude of notes I wrote while I had the tube in my mouth and could not talk. These are not necessarily in any particular order. I include it to show what was happening in real time.
Go (for) your run
I'm so tired
No tube out
Is it normal to have tube for 3 days
Do you need to clean your house (to Lori)
Sorry (it took) so long
Could to? Check with my ?? – in still way
Yoppy happy thanks for everything
I don't feel strong
Are my teeth broken
Are they giving me a bath
Boo
Sat X, Sun X, Mon – maybe (re tube)
Shit
Thanks so much
Lori saw my incision
I still getting the blue sleeping pill?
How bad do I look?
Strong sleeping pill - When?
Pain killer soon?
Call Lori to bring brush and curling iron
What sleeping pill do I get?
They work
This is tougher than before
Tomorrow tube?
Rob and A get home?

When they brush my teeth, I get moisture
Pain with breathing tube
I am alive
December 10
How sexy!! (in reference to wiping drool)
Bum (sore from sitting)
What are the breathing numbers – 28, 99
Tell the doctor I have the tube in for 6 days – no fair!!
Is the operation a success – Am I going to be an
invalid
Put ice in the jar. Thanks for letting me use and for
letting Lori to the dry mouth department
You saw me at my worst last night
How often can I have my mouth watered?
Every half hour Lori gave me a mouth wash of ice
water
Should I rest. What's next
Irritation, irritation
Sharp spots on tongue
Food tubes? What the hell?
When will I have fluid, ice
It hurts to pee
Great to see Grant
Sorry Lori for having you see me choke – it hurts
Brush teeth
Pain in the chest
Ice
My tongue is raw
My blue pill at 10
My mouth dry
Thank you for putting up with me last night
Sorry thanks for being here
Can't breathe
Thank God for you 2

I will need a total hair treatment
When do I rest
When can I get in bed and Tylenol
You missed the first doctor – this is different
My husband is coming at 9
Is my husband here
Please is it OK for Brian to stay while you change
bandages
I just wanted him to see my scars
Can't breathe – what time
Phone – I could text you
Plan tomorrow – you have your workout – be here by
10 = Lori at 12 – you nap, run you come back at 4 –
Lori 8 to 10
She (Lori) wants to be here – she is working while
here a little. But that's important to talk to her about
enough time for work
Go for your run
I'm so tired
When was that? I had terrible dreams
So glad you were here
Worse last night – couldn't catch my breath
I feel like such a pain in the neck for you and Lori –
just a drain
I really need you – don't give up on me
You look good
Workout, rest, run, come back
I need to sleep
Sleeping 9:30 – really tired
When I've had my heart pill, go home, rest
When can I have my sleeping pill
Please, pain killer
My bum is sore. When the nurse comes back ask if I
can sit on the edge of the bed

Is there hockey tonight

Re: BAD NURSE (I wasn't happy with one particular nurse)
Can't make enemies – we need her – I'll play the game right now – I never want to see her again
Useless, ass, tit – slow, doesn't listen (referring to nurse)
Missed the doctors ask her what they said
Tell Lori to be careful, we need friends

Re: BAD NIGHT
Didn't sleep last night – soap opera going on
Long story, tell you when I can
Come here to chase doctors
In the bed – drunk, police, noise
Finally they put my bed back and gave me a 2nd pill
I woke up in the dark – pushed my bed – nurses behind me
Are people talking about last night? I'm sure a nurse was sent home – fired?
I woke up thought I died – nurse came by said we have trouble – a new admission problem
Drug – abused her – boyfriend cam in – refused care and drug
I asked – boy swinging his stethoscope - Devil admitting people
I have terrible dreams - devil

Re: TUBE REMOVAL
Pretty scary – five or six doctors came running – I had the best nurse last night
I'm still here!
The best nurse

You saved my life
I'm scared - sounds pretty bad this morning – code
blue
I think I was almost a goner - scary
Ice cold face cloth – wash face – can I have a cold
water flush in my mouth
When can I be fed ice
Big day today – hopefully no steps backward
Don't leave until the doctors come back – not until
the doctors decide what they do next
Can I sit with my legs over the bed with pillows
supporting?
Come to hear doctor – I want you to here whenever
he shows up

Appendix C

Texts and Emails – December 2017

Following are the majority of the texts sent and received by Brian during the hospital process. Most of them are with Lori and Rob, but several are with Brian's sons, Tony and Cam. Some are friends - Wayne, Loretta, Marlene, Dot. Also, there are several interchanges with our family Doctor - Dr. Schaub who followed my journey throughout.

To Dr. Schaub Nov 27
Rochelle will be admitted Sunday Dec 3. She is to stop warfarin on Thursday Nov 30. Operation is all day Tues Dec 5.
To Lori Dec 3 3:31 pm
Just in case it didn't come through it's unit 9-1 room 28 bed B
To Lori Dec 3 4:51 pm
Going for xray. Took blood already. Should start heparin soon. She will be ready for early night.
To Lori Dec 3 5:03 pm
Supper served. But we didn't tell them we had a greasy burger and fries while waiting for the bed.
To Lori Dec 3 5:06 pm
With activities happening her mind is occupied and she is focused and doing well. Tomorrow should be a lite day with lots of opportunity for visiting and wandering.
To Lori Dec 3 5:10 pm

Surgery set for 10:30 Tues. There is a waiting room for family with a direct line to the nurse. Once in ICU visitors are allowed but we might not be able to communicate. After ICU there is a couple of days in post ICU with visitors allowed. Then back to ward for recovery.

To Cam Dec 4 10:41am

All is well. Just in a holding pattern until surgery tomorrow at 10:30. Prepping the blood and continuing with meds. Rochelle is in good spirits and feeling positive. It feels like a competent environment with everyone knowing what to do.

To Cam Dec 4 10:50am

Yesterday was a tough day with Rochelle having the "what if" talk with Lori and Rob.

To Cam Dec 4 11:03am

Just met with surgeon. Start at 1pm tomorrow. He is quite positive. 6 hour operation.

To Cam Dec 4 1:00 pm

Just met with surgeon. Start at 1pm tomorrow. He is quite positive. 6 hour operation.

From Dr Schaub Dec 4 4:33pm

Hi Brian, is Rochelle admitted to hospital now?

To Dr. Schaub Dec 4 4:43pm

Got in last night. On heparin substitute. Operation at 1pm tomorrow. Dr Kidd is confident. All is well.

To Loretta Dec 5 9:34 am

Thanks so much. Operation at 1pm about 5 to 6 hrs. Surgeon is quite upbeat. Excellent care here. Will keep everyone posted.

To Marlene and Cam Dec 5 12:35 pm

She's in the operating room

To Lori Dec 5 12:36 pm

She's drugged and relaxed. Calm and positive

From Lori Dec 5 12:36 pm
Are you staying at the hospital ?
To Lori Dec 5 12:38 pm
No. I'm heading home to rest. Will be back around 4pm
From Lori Dec 5 12:38 pm
Ok. We will be there shortly after 5
From Lori Dec 5 4:36 pm
Are you there ?
To Lori Dec 5 4:36 pm
Yes. Sitting in the family room. All quiet. No word yet.
Email to Tony Dec 5 8:52 pm
Rochelle is out if surgery and in ICU. Will see her soon but she will be under for a couple of days. Operation went ok but not perfect. They haven't closed her chest yet due to bleeding. Hopefully they can get it done by Thursday.
Will keep you posted.
To Dr Shaub Dec 5 10:17pm
Rochelle made it through surgery. Some complications but stable. In ICU with her chest still open due to bleeding. Dr. Kidd thinks she will be ok but may take a couple days to close her up and wake her.
To Rob and Lori - Dec 6 6:16 am
Called ICU. She had a good night. Still heavily sedated but they have backed off on some meds. Minimal bleeding. Sounds ok.
To Cam Dec 6 8:36am
She had a good night. Still sedated with chest open. Seeing the doctor in an hour to discuss next step
From Lori Dec 6 8:47 am

How are you holding up?
To Lori Dec 6 8:48 am
Hanging in. On my way to the hospital
From Lori Dec 6 8:51 am
Brian. I wanted to apologize. Through all this none of us have asked how YOU are doing. Grant was very quick to point that out this morning. You told Rob yesterday that Anika is the light of my moms life and I know she is one of the lights in yours. Am sorry that we as a family have all been very selfish and in our own heads as to what this all means individually. We will see you soon.
To Lori Dec 6 9:09 am
No problem. Don't worry about it. We all need to deal on our own way. Just arrived at the hospital.
From Lori Dec 6 9:14 am
Annalise is staying with the baby and grant has a meeting so it might just be Rob and I
To Lori Dec 6 9:31 am
Just visited with her. Not much change. Other than puffiness she looks ok. Doctors were into see her earlier and making a plan. Just in the family room now waiting for the doctor.
To Marlene and Cam Dec 6 5:39 pm
At the hospital. They will take her back to the OR in a couple hours and see if they can close her up. If so the will start to wake her late tonight. So far all is well but we are still in the critical phase.
From Dr Schaub Dec 6 6:03 pm
Thank you for the update Brian. Wishing her a good recovery.
To Rob and Lori - Dec 6 7:09 pm

Still not in OR yet. Family room is full of people waiting for word. Likely won't go in until these folks get notified about their relatives.

To Lori Dec 6 8:07 pm

No visiting now until after 8:30. If nothing by then I will go to ICU to see her and talk with nurse.

To Rob and Lori - Dec 6 8:58 pm

She was scheduled to go next but one of her roommates had an emergency reentry to OR. Depends on how long that one takes so it may wait until morning. They suggested I go home and call in the morning. They have my number if there are any problems but she seems to be doing well.

To Marlene and Cam Dec 6 9:42 pm

She got preempted due to an emergency. She may get in tonight or maybe not until morning. They told me to go home and call them in the morning.

To Marlene and Cam Dec 6 10:08 pm

Home now. Rochelle is stable. Bleeding is under control. Will talk to doctor in the morning.

To Rob and Lori Dec 6 11:28 pm

Just got a call from Dr Kidd. She is back together and all is well. They will start waking her up in the morning. I will call first thing and see how it's going and let you know.

To Marlene and Cam Dec 6 11:33 pm

Just got a call from the surgeon. Rochelle is back together and all is well. They will start waking her in the morning. I will call first thing and see how it's going.

To Rob and Lori Dec 7 6:12 am

Called ICU. They are starting to bring her out. Not alert yet. They suggest not to come until after shift change. Maybe around 9. There was some bleeding but it has stopped. Legs are jerky but she is always like that. Tubes still in. I will head up around 8 to be there just after shift change.

To Rob and Lori Dec 7 8:49 am

Still haven't got in to see her. Looks like they are telling all visitors to hold off. Sounds like a staff issue not a patient issue.

To Loretta Dec 7 10:00 am

She is waking up. Still with tubes so she's not happy. But doing well. Still in ICU

To Marlene and Cam Dec 7 11:32 am

She is awake now. Not fully alert. Still has the breathing tube which is driver her nuts. Hopefully that will come out later today. She is quite uncomfortable.

To Wayne Dec 7 3:41pm

Rochelle is awake but uncomfortable with tubes everywhere. Can't communicate yet. Still in ICU for a few days.

To Rob and Lori Dec 7 9:03 am

I'm in. Any time us good. She's starting to wake and looks confused and stressed. Tubes still in.

To Rob and Lori Dec 7 3:16 pm

No change. Tubes still in. She hates it and is very uncomfortable. Not sure if it will be out today.

To Lori Dec 7 3:54 pm

Bloodwork is fine. She couldn't handle the extra load of breathing as they turned down the machine. So they turned it back up.

From Lori Dec 7 3:54 pm

Oh okay. When the doctor was in the morning he wasn't happy with the blood flow and that is why he said they couldn't take it out.

From Lori Dec 7 3:58 pm

Am sending Rob and Annalise. I am not coming.

To Lori Dec 7 4:40 pm

Rob and Anna are in now. Your mom is much more alert and aware. But not very happy. No pain but very uncomfortable. Doctor hope the tube can come out tomorrow. No comment on blood flow so that must be ok. Just needs to demonstrate more independent breathing. They keep testing by lowering the assist.

From Lori Dec 7 4:45 pm

Ok. I'll come in the morning and Anna is keeping the baby at home.

To Franci Dec 7 9:11pm

It's been a rough couple of days. She had her operation Tuesday. It went ok but a couple of glitches the meant they kept her under with her chest open. Late last night they were able to close her chest. This morning they allowed her to start waking up. But she still has lots of tubes and wires making her quite uncomfortable. Hopefully tomorrow they will take the tube from her throat. Will keep you posted.

To Rob and Lori Dec 8 5:51 am

Called ICU. She had a good night. Tube still in. They will assess at doctor's rounds. I'm going up about 9.

To Marlene and Cam Dec 8 10:59 am

Not much change. She is alert but tube still in. So communicating is difficult. No sign of tube coming out any time soon. All other indicators are good.

To Lori Dec 8 4:15 pm

Sound asleep right now. Tube still in. Looks like they reduced the assist. Still breathing too rapidly.

To Rob Dec 8 6:50 pm

Sounds good. Shift change should be over by 8:30. I'm leaving in about 10 minutes. No real change. All are hoping to get the tube out tomorrow but no promises. She is sleeping off and on but quite alert when awake.

From Rob Dec 8 9:37 pm

It was a good visit, she could hold a pencil to write.

To Rob and Lori Dec 9 6:610 am

Called ICU. Everything about the same. Good sleep. No pain. Tolerating tube. Will decide on tube later today. I will be up there after shift change.

To Rob and Lori Dec 9 9:43 am

Much the same. Not much progress on getting rid tube. Likely not today physio here now. Was some fluid around the lungs yesterday. She is writing notes. Not feeling very happy right now.

To Marlene and Cam Dec 9 5:05 pm

Still in ICU with tube. Probably a couple more days. She is strong but not happy. I plan on coming to the game tomorrow. Lori will be with her mom then.

From Rob Dec 9 9:55 am

Good she can communicate. But shitty that its going slower... we got thru security and will have a tough time getting back w baby. But will be nice to get home

To Lori Dec 9 5:56 pm

I'm here for another hour or so. She is up and in the chair after another workout. She wants you to bring a brush and curling iron tomorrow. I tried helping with her hair but I'm hopeless.

To Rob Dec 9 1:06 pm

Good to hear. Your mom is having lots of activity today. Physio bath etc. She is worn out. Tube in for another day or two.

To Lori Dec 9 7:10 pm

Shift change. Heading home now. She has been in the chair for a couple of hours. Ready to get back in her bed and get a sleeping pill and pain killer (mouth). Hutterite ladies asked how my daughter (Rochelle) is doing. Do I look that old?

To Rob Dec 9 7:57 pm

Between Lori and me your mom was covered all day. A couple of physio sessions and cleaning. She was up in a chair a couple of times for several hours each time. Still has the tube. Likely not out til Monday. No pain other than with the tube. Getting stronger gradually but gets tired. More tomorrow.

To Rob and Lori Dec 10 9:03 am

She seems tired and a bit less alert. But she had a heavy sleeping pill so may not be fully awake yet. Some pain in throat from tube. Had some painkillers for that. Some improvement in breathing. They are testing right now to see how she's doing. There is a chance the tube could come out later today but I'm not optimistic. But likely tomorrow.

To Rob and Lori Dec 10 9:05 am

Fluid is down a litre with lasix. Fluid around the lung is down slightly.

From Lori Dec 10 11:18 am

Have the doctors been in yet?

To Lori Dec 10 11:21 am

They were in first thing and were testing her breathing. They hadn't returned to check the results by the time I left. I'm out at Cain's game and will be back to the hospital right after.

To Rob Dec 10 2:09 pm
All indicators are moving in the right direction but very slowly. They will give her another physio workout in an hour and will adjust her breathing assist as a test. She might be ready for tube removal tonight but would wait until morning at the earliest. She has had some chest pain but likely at the incision/bone.

To Franci Dec 10 8:21 pm
Still in ICU with a breathing tube and other assorted wires. She is alert and communicating with notes. Hopefully the tube can come out tomorrow. She is quite uncomfortable but no pain other than due to the tube. The operation itself was good but a long recovery ahead.

To Rob and Lori - Dec 11 8:46 am
Breathing rate is higher. She seems a bit stressed and anxious. Not good signs for tube removal. Doctors and techs will be around later and hopefully we will get a better assessment. She seems tired.

From Lori Dec 11 8:46 am
Did she sleep?

To Lori Dec 11 8:48 am
Not a good sleep

From Lori Dec 11 8:49 am
When you say the breathing is higher you mean stronger or that she is breathing too fast like yesterday?

To Lori Dec 11 8:49 am
Too fast. It is at or above 40 when she was below 30. HR is high. Up to 99. I'd say today is a backwards day so far. We'll see how it goes. Doing rounds now.

From Lori Dec 11 8:54 am

Ok let me know. Dammit. She needs to sleep. They should have made sure that happened.
From Lori Dec 11 8:55 am
I know she knows this but if she can relax the tube will come out.
From Lori Dec 11 9:02 am
Please let me know what the doctors say. I plan to be there for 1pm. But can come sooner.
To Lori Dec 11 9:13 am
No tube removal today. Some progress but not enough. Removal would put too much strain on the heart.
From Lori Dec 11 9:17 am
Ok. Is she ok? What about the chest tubes?
To Lori Dec 11 9:17 am
Physically yes. But not happy.
To Lori Dec 11 9:18 am
No other tubes removed.
From Lori Dec 11 9:20 am
Well at least that is something positive she can focus on.
To Lori Dec 11 9:38 am
Breathing test much the same as yesterday. They focus on frequency and volume. Assisted frequency is below 30 but above 40 on test. Too high. Volume is 300 on assist but 100 on test. Too low.
To Wayne Dec 11 9:46 am
Still in ICU with breathing tube. Alert but not happy. Progress but slow.
To Lori Dec 11 12:12 pm

Everything about the same. I got kicked out with another patient's procedure. Sounds like they might be taking out some chest tubes now. Hopefully I can get back in after 15 minutes.

To Lori Dec 11 12:16 pm

I will stay until you get here and then take a break for run and lunch. Then I will come back until evening shift change.

From Lori Dec 11 12:17 pm

Ok. I'll be there in an hour and will come back after 8:30pm for her bedtime. How are her spirits?

To Lori Dec 11 12:18 pm

Not great. She looks depressed.

To Lori Dec 11 10:02 am

Kidd stopped by and chatted. Quite sad that the tube is still in but not his call. He is happy with heart progress. He is off hospital duty this week but will get associate to stop by.

To Rob Dec 11 10:58 am

Tube will not come out today. Lungs not strong enough. Doing regular physio and spending most of the day in a chair. Removing chest tubes and putting her in bed for a couple hours. Kidd stopped by and is pleased with the heart progress.

To Rob Dec 11 11:01 am

They don't want to risk removing the breathing tube and have to put it back in. But she is quite down because of it.

Email to Tony Dec 11 12:02 pm

Just to keep you updated.

Rochelle is still in ICU with breathing tube. She is alert and can write notes. She wants off the tube but her lungs are not strong enough yet. Hopefully in a day or two. Heart function seems good. Long recovery ahead.

To Marlene and Cam Dec 11 12:03 pm

Still on the breathing tube. Progress is slow. Maybe tomorrow but I wouldn't count on it. She is not happy.

To Rob Dec 11 4:46 pm

Looking brighter this afternoon. Had a couple of physio sessions including some walking and step ups at the bedside. Breathing tests show modest improvement. I doubt it is enough to get the tube out tomorrow. Better spirits but frustrated.

To Rob and Lori Dec 11 7:00 pm

Shift change. Just leaving. She is quite alert and looking good. She had another breathing test and I thought the numbers looked impressive. The tech said it was modest improvement and didn't indicate we were any closer to tube removal. She is tired and looking forward to a better night's sleep.

To Dr Shaub Dec 11 7:03 pm

Almost a week since surgery. She is making progress but still in ICU with a breathing tube. She is quite alert and can write notes. She is anxious to have the tube removed but her lungs are not yet strong enough. Hopefully in the next day or two.

To Rob and Lori Dec 11 7:03 pm

Shift change. Leaving now. Breathing test went well. They are still talking about removing tube tomorrow but I will believe it when I see it. She will get a painkiller and sleeping pill before 10.

From Dr Shaub Dec 11 7:17 pm

Thank you Brian. I did look on netcare to see her progress over the last days. I hope they are able to keep her comfortable in the meantime. Wishing you both all the best and Rochelle strength during her recovery.

From Lori Dec 11 10:22 pm

Still here. Will leave when the nurse comes back from break and gives her a sleeping pill. Is pretty quite here so far and have closed her drape so nice and dark. She is resting now. They were doing another breathing test when I came and it was very difficult for her so think she is pretty tired.

To Lori Dec 12 8:59 am

Can you be here for 10 am meeting with doctor

To Lori Dec 12 9:05 am

Making progress but wants to give us a full update

From Lori Dec 12 9:22 am

Her spirits? That is what am worried about.

To Lori Dec 12 9:23 am

She's ok but not great. More pissed off with nurse than anything.

From Lori Dec 12 9:24 am

The night one? Or her new one today?

To Lori Dec 12 9:25 am

The same day nurse as yesterday. She is a pain.

From Lori Dec 12 9:25 am

Oh yeah

To Lori Dec 12 9:26 am

She gets annoyed at everything especially questions from family. She would be happy if family stayed home.

From Lori Dec 12 9:27 am

Well too bad for her.

From Lori Dec 12 9:27 am

The night one was old school as well but willing to listen and walked me through everything. I was there till after midnight and she thanked me for being there.

To Lori Dec 12 9:28 am

I think she is my age or older. Should be retired.

From Lori Dec 12 9:28 am

Yup and not in that industry.

From Lori Dec 12 12:24 pm

Can you bring her glasses and her reading tablet when you come back. Thanks

To Lori Dec 12 2:56 pm

She froze me out again. Likes control. Hopefully another 10 minutes.

From Lori Dec 12 2:57 pm

No that is not it Brain and change that attitude or it won't get better.

From Lori Dec 12 2:58 pm

I had a long talk with her nurse and she was almost in tears. She is good.

From Lori Dec 12 2:59 pm

Dont come in with that attitude.

From Lori Dec 12 3:07 pm

Brian she is getting an ECG. They will let you in as soon as done.   You keeping calling is upsetting her and the nurses and is why the doctors had to talk to us this morning.

From Lori Dec 12 3:18 pm

They are done now. Not sure if you got the call.

To Rob Dec 12 5:43 pm

Not much new. She had a bad night last night but is doing well today. Had a brief meeting with doctors today. They are happy with progress but it is slow. Tube will be in for a while as her lungs strengthen. She is in ok spirits.

To Lori Dec 12 7:02 pm

They are just putting her into bed. Did over 2.5 hours on test. Handled it well but was tired towards the end. Shift change now.

To Loretta Dec 13 7:55am

Thanks for the note. She is still in ICU with a breathing tube and other assorted wires. But she is improving.

To Rob and Lori - Dec 13 9:02 am

Tube is out. Mask is on. She coughed the tube out herself causing a major panic on the ward. She is doing well on the mask but they will do some testing this morning. They hope not but there is a chance the tube will have to go back in.

To Cam Dec 13 9:47am

She is getting some assist with the mask but is doing fine.

To Marlene and Cam Dec 13 9:45 am

Breathing tube is finally out and she is on a mask. She coughed out the tube causing an emergency and panic. But she seems fine now. Hopefully they don't have to put the tube back in.

To Cam Dec 13 9:56am

No talking yet. Mask and irritated throat

To Rob and Lori Dec 13 10:39 am

Mask off for now. Will likely go back on later but retubing looks unlikely. Doing physio now.

From Lori Dec 13 7:28 am

I stayed till about midnight. Her numbers were the best I have seen. Low 20's high 300's for the breathing, heart rate constant as well as oxidation. Her blood pressure fell and they were watching it. They didn't give her a sleeping pill because of what happened the night before but did give her the pain pill. She seemed to be sleeping good when left and was in good spirits when awake.

From Lori Dec 13 9:18 am

How is she?

To Lori Dec 13 9:19 am

Happy. But the incident was pretty scary.

To Lori Dec 13 9:21 am

Sounds like it happened during or just before shift change. Doctors came. Will be doing rounds soon and hope to get assessment. Looks ok and the nurses and techs are happy.

From Lori Dec 13 9:23 am

Ok because yesterday the doctors said they weren't sure she would survive the procedure of having to put the tube back in. Please let me know what the doctors say.

From Lori Dec 13 10:05 am

Ask if the heart flutter has corrected itself.

To Lori Dec 13 10:08 am

Sounds like it was there to a minor extent but ok now. The tube incident was major. The doctor said it was a close call. Haven't done official rounds yet.

From Lori Dec 13 10:09 am

Ok. Should I come now? Yes I know. They were very clear in the meeting that they are not sure she can survive the procedure of putting it back in if that have too.

To Lori Dec 13 10:11 am
She's doing exceptionally well now. No rush to come in. She is happy doctor is happy nurse is happy
From Lori Dec 13 11:13 am
Can she talk?
To Lori Dec 13 11:16 am
Hoarse whisper. Best she doesn't talk much yet. Will get ice chips soon. She's excited for that.
To Lori Dec 13 1:11 pm
They are just putting in a nose tube for meds an nutrition. They don't think she's ready to swallow. I had to leave while the do it so I will take off until around 4. Make sure you call to get entry.
To Marlene Dec 13 5:54pm
Sorry. I'm in the icu. Everything is going well. Major crisis at 8am. It was an emergency and it was close. But she is doing great now. No tube no mask. She has even eaten some pudding.
To Lori Dec 13 7:06 pm
Shift change. Leaving now. Doing great. Needs to work on exercises for her lung capacity. The plastic device by the bed and breathing exercises on the paper by the window.
To Lori Dec 14 9:09 am
Still not in. But I talked to her on the phone. She is getting ready to move to unit 91. She sounds great.
To Marlene and Cam Dec 14 9:15 am
Haven't been able to get in to see Rochelle yet. They won't let me in. But they did let me talk to her on the phone. She sounds great and they are getting her ready to leave ICU and go to the ward. Good news.
To Rob Dec 14 9:14 am

Haven't seen your mom yet. They haven't let me in. But I talked to her on the phone and she sounds great. They are just getting her ready to move out of ICU and into the ward. That's good news.

To Lori Dec 14 9:54 am

In 936 unit 91. This is a drop-down room. 2 to 3 days in here then move to a ward room. No calling required to visit. No visitors between 12:30 and 2:30. I will stay til 12:30 then come back by 4:30.   She had a good night and looks great. I can get back after about 15 minutes of prep.

To Rob Dec 14 9:56 am

She is in the step down unit. A couple days here and then to the ward. She looks and feels great.

To Lori Dec 14 10:25 am

She's settled in. Made one trip to the toilet on her own. Nurse and assistant took her for a long walk to the weigh scale and back. 48.1 kg. Up from under 40 on admission. No oxygen needed.

To Marlene and Cam Dec 14 10:35 am

Now out of ICU. Off oxygen. Still lots of IVs. Went for a long walk with nurse. Still lots of fluid in her system. Doing well but tired and weak.

To Rob and Lori Dec 14 11:11 am

Had physio did well. Not much info from doctor at rounds. Will assess later today. No sign of retubing. Plan on keeping mask ready if needed. May put it on at night. The incident was at 8am but recovered very quickly.

To Dorothy Dec 14 12:09pm

Thanks. Big progress in the last 24 hours. We should be out of the critical phase and into the recovery phase.

To Lori Dec 14 12:19 pm
Leaving shortly. She is exhausted from all the excitement and is finally sleeping. She took all her pills orally. Therapist and speech person (check on throat after so many days on tube) will be around sometime today.

From Lori Dec 14 4:06 pm
Yeah totally. And had to go get her a Coke Zero. First thing she wanted when they cleared her to eat with no restrictions now.

To Lori Dec 14 7:08 pm
Just getting ready to leave. She is getting some help to the toilet then plans on resting. She had been having deep restful sleeps so hopefully she will sleep all night. They say this ward is much quieter than ICU so that will help.

To Rob and Lori Dec 15 9:04 am
Hi Rob and Lori. Your mom had a good night and is still progressing well. Now that she is somewhat mobile and can communicate verbally and by text I won't provide regular updates. She will stay in communication with you. All looks good but still a long road ahead.

To Wayne Dec 15 9:21am
Out of ICU. Looking good. We should now be out of the critical phase and into recovery. Long way to go yet.

To Loretta and Dot Dec 15 9:30am
To the Adamaches and Echtners. First full day in post ICU. All is well starting to remove some of the wires and tubes. Occasional use of oxygen via loose nose strap. A couple of days here then to a regular ward to work on rehab and recovery.

To Dr Shaub Dec 15 9:31am

All is well. Out of ICU and hopefully into recovery mode then rehab. She is feeling good. Still a long road ahead.

To Franci Dec 15 9:34 am

Out of ICU. Off oxygen for the most part. Still other tubes and wires. Feeling good so hopefully we can now start the long recovery.

Email to Tony Dec 15 9:52 am

Hi Tony

Rochelle is now out of ICU and off breathing tubes. She is feeling great. Hopefully we can now move to the long recovery phase.

To Cam Dec 16 10:43 am

Rochelle is making progress. We have been for a couple walks. Still lots of fluid but reducing slowly. Needs oxygen as her lungs are still not strong enough. We take it off for the walks. She has no food restrictions but has a limited appetite. We are pleased with the progress .

To Marlene and Cam Dec 18 12:21 pm

Just removing the last attachment. Then she should be free of any tubes and wires. May put on another drip temporarily. She is walking several times a day and eating reasonably well. Looking good.

To Lori Dec 20 10:49 am

(weight) Down but not much. They are increasing lasix to 90 twice daily. By injection not drip.

To Lori Dec 21 11:44 am

Moved to 28-1. End of the other hall. Same room as when she came in Dec 3. Has gone for an angiogram but not the invasive kind.

To Rob Dec 21 11:55 am

She's been moved out of post ICU to a regular ward. Just took her away for an angiogram. Still working on getting rid of fluids. Will try to drain fluid around the lungs tomorrow. Walking and moving well but short of breath due to fluid.
To Lori Dec 21 11:57 am
She is too well to be in those rooms and they needed her bed for an ICU discharge.
To Lori Dec 21 11:58 am
Not sure why they called for angiogram. We weren't expecting it. Dr Kidd didn't mention anything yesterday.
To Lori Dec 21 11:59 am
There are no visiting restrictions in the ward. No mandatory rest times.
To Marlene Dec 21 12:51pm
Rochelle has been moved to the regular ward. Means they think she needs less attention. Still lots if fluid to get rid of. Will try draining fluid around her lungs which makes her winded when walking. Some progress each day but it will still be a long haul.
To Franci Dec 23 7:28pm
She's made really good progress. They are trying to send her home in the next couple of days but we want to make sure she's ready. She is still weak but walking well and did stairs today with physio. Still some fluid retention but much better. All is looking positive so hopefully just a long recovery period.
To Dr Shaub Dec 24 12:24pm
Rochelle is being discharged today. She is doing remarkably well with some residual swelling. Will make an appointment with you into the new year. Merry Christmas to you.
From Dr Shaub Dec 24 12:38 pm

Hi Brian, thank you for the message. That's great news. Wishing you both a Merry Xmas and a good start to the New Year. I will be back at work on the 2nd, please feel free to contact me otherwise I will see you both soon.

To Marlene and Cam Dec 24 2:25 pm

She's home

To Wayne Dec 24 2:33pm

She's home. Recovery is going faster than expected. They sent her home today. Tired and weak but happy to be home.

To Franci Dec 24 2:34pm

Rochelle is home. Tired and weak but happy to be home. Recovery is progressing.

To Loretta and Dot Dec 24 2:38pm

Rochelle is recovering faster than expected. They sent her home today. Tired and weak but happy to be home. Still a long recovery ahead.

Email to Tony Dec 24 2:41 pm

Hi Tony

Rochelle is recovering faster than expected and they sent her home today. Tired and weak but happy to be home. Still a long road ahead.

To Dr Shaub Dec 28

You may be aware that Rochelle was discharged on Dec 24. She is doing well and has shed most of her fluids and is now at her preoperative weight. She had bloodwork done this morning so I called Medical Express to see if someone might give us the results. They said that you would be checking the system while away. If so can you call or text the results. Otherwise can you give us someone to call at the clinic. Thanks.

From Dr Shaub Dec 28
Results don't come back for a good day. I looked them up on netcare, all labs are normal but inr is a bit low. Are you free for a call?

Appendix D
March 2017 Angiogram

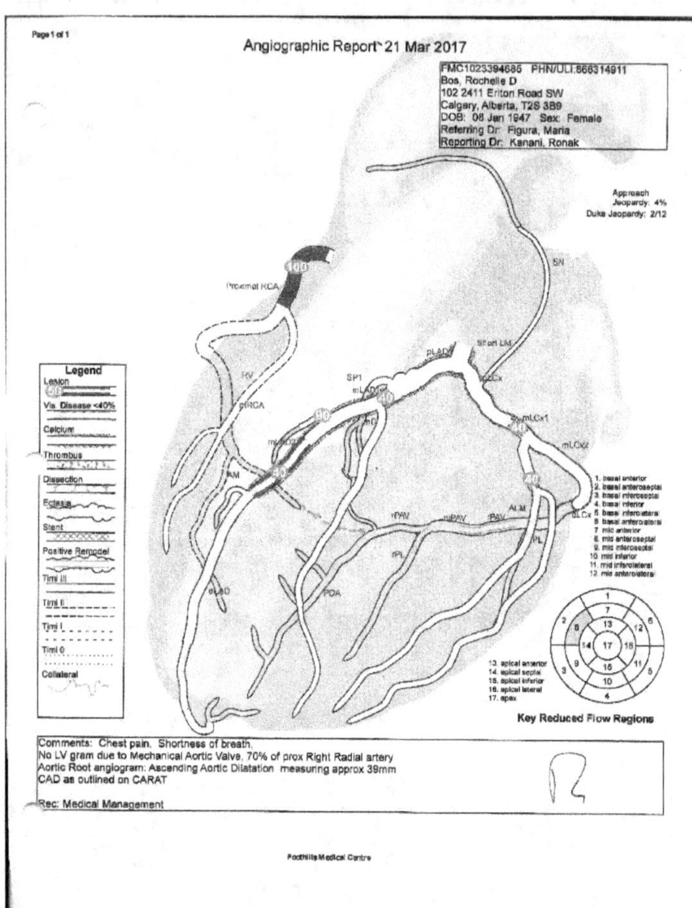

Appendix E
March 2017 Discharge

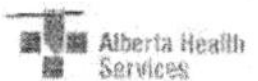

Alberta Health Services	**Discharge Summary - Cardiac Sciences**	**CONFIDENTIAL**

Patient Name: Bos, Rochelle D   **Gender:** Female   **Confidentiality:**

RHRN: 1023304688   **ULI:** 866314911   **Age:** 70y   **DOB:** 1947-Jan-08   **Service:** Cardio

Visit/Enc ID: 10004168816   **Adm/Reg Date:** 2017-Mar-17   **Attending MD:** Abdi Ali, Ahmed

Location: FMC-81-834-4

Document Created: 2017-Mar-24 By: Quevillon, Joey (Medical Student)

Visit Data

- **Admit Date:** 2017-Mar-17
- **Discharge Date:** 2017-Mar-28
- **Discharged From:** Foothills Medical Centre (FMC-81)

Goals of Care

- **Goals of Care:**
  Goals of Care Designation R1. Designation Definition: Patient is expected to benefit from and is accepting of any appropriate investigations/interventions that can be offered including attempted resuscitation and ICU care. This GCD has been ordered after relevant conversation with the patient.

Allergy and Intolerances

Allergies

- **No Known Allergies**

Cardiac Risk Factors

- **Modifiable:** Dyslipidemia

Diagnosis

- **Admitting Dx:** CHF, Chest Pain, Query Unstable Angina, CHF, Chest Pain, Query Unstable Angina

Diagnostic Imaging / Cardiovascular Labs

- **ECG:** Electrocardiogram
- **ECG:** Electrocardiogram
- **ECG:** Electrocardiogram
- **ECG:** Electrocardiogram
- **ECG:** Electrocardiogram
- **ECG:** Electrocardiogram
- **General Radiology:** GR Chest, 2 Projections
- **General Radiology:** GR Chest, 2 Projections
- **ECG:** Electrocardiogram
- **ECG:** Electrocardiogram

Interventions

- **Interventions:**
  Angiogram (right and/or left heart cath). 2017-Mar-21. Coronary/LV Angiogram ---------------------- 100% pRCA (with collaterals) 40% mLAD 40% LCx/OM.

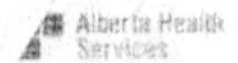

Alberta Health Services

Discharge Summary - Cardiac Sciences

Patient Name: Bos, Rochelle D				Gender: Female	Confidentiality:
RHRN: 1023394685	ULI: 866314911	Age: 70y	DOB: 1947-Jan-08	Service: Cardio	
Visit/Enc ID: 106044168816	Adm/Reg Date: 2017-Mar-17		Attending MD: Abdi Ali, Ahmed		
Location: FMC-81-834-4					

Document Created: 2017-Mar-24 By: Quevillon, Joey (Medical Student)

Course In Hospital

MOST RESPONSIBLE DIAGNOSIS: Unstable angina and CHF

PROFILE:
1. Congenital bicuspid aortic valve - bioprosthetic valve replacement (1982), mechanical valve replacement 1996 (Regina). On warfarin, target INR 2.5-3.5. Primary cardiologist Dr Kanani.
2. Echo Feb 2017 - moderate LV systolic dysfunction, mild-moderate MR, severe TR, mean gradient (aortic valve) 11, peak gradient 24.
3. Permanent pacemaker
4. Dyslipidemia - LDL 3.5 Mar 2017
5. Sigmoid polyps

SOCIAL HISTORY: Married. Non-smoker. Retired teacher.

HPI: Patient presented to ED with a 1 week history of worsening SOBOE and chest tightness. An echo done early in the week (Total Cardiology) shows worsening EF (moderate LV dysfunction) and well seated mechanical aortic valve with normal gradients. She had mildly elevated troponin (44) and her NT-pro BNP was 3205.

She was admitted to Cardiology for management of unstable angina and mild congestive heart failure.

ISSUES IN HOSPITAL:
1) Unstable angina/CAD: An angiogram was completed and showed chronic 100% occlusion of her pRCA with collaterals and mild disease (40%) in her mLAD and LCx/OM. The recommendation was for medical management. She was started on ASA 81mg, bisoprolol, perindopril, atorvastatin. Due to her high LDL of 3.5, ezetimibe was added in addition to the statin. She did have a mild elevation in her liver enzymes (ALT 47) which should be monitored in context of her ongoing statin use.

2) Congestive heart failure: She was diuresed with Lasix and started on a nitro patch. She was clinically euvolemic at discharge. See above for the cardiac medications initiated in hospital.

3) Mechanical Aortic valve: Her aortic valve was well seated with normal gradients on her recent echocardiogram (TotalCardiology-report from this year). Her warfarin was stopped and she was on IV heparin in hospital for completion of her angiogram. Prior to discharge home, her warfarin was re-started and her INR was 3.6 on March 28 upon discharge. She will be discharged on warfarin 3mg PO daily for Tuesday march 28 and Wednesday March 29. She will get her INR checked on March 29 and her family physician Dr Schaub will follow up on these results and direct further dosing modifications based on her INR. Dr Schaub will continue with her outpatient warfarin monitoring.

4) Shoulder Pain: Patient complained of a new onset (2 weeks before presentation) of Right Shoulder pain. She doesn't seem to find a link between it's pain and the chest tightness and it did not respond to Nitro. It sounds likely MSK related and physio can be looked at as an outpatient option.

Discharge Summary - Cardiac Sciences **CONFIDENTIAL**

Patient Name: Bos, Rochelle D Gender: Female Confidentiality:

RLRN: 1023394685 ULI: 86631491 Age: 70y DOB: 1947-Jan-08 Service: Cardio

Visit/Enc ID: 100044168816 Adm/Reg.Date: 2017-Mar-17 Attending MD: Abdi Ali, Ahmed

Location: FMC-81-834-4

Document Created: 2017-Mar-24 By: Quevillon, Joey (Medical Student)

Completion

- Summary Complete: .

Patient Height, Weight, BMI

- **Weight kg:** 43.6

- **Weight was documented:** 2017-Mar-28

Electronic Signatures:

Abdi Ali, Ahmed (MD-Cardiology)

*Authored:*Completion,Vaccinations and Blood Products Administered,Follow-up and Recommendations,Events of Hospital Stay,Medications,Copies,Patient Height, Weight, BMI

Figura, Maria (MD-Cardiology) (Signed 2017-Mar-27 9:30)

*Authored:*Vaccinations and Blood Products Administered,Diagnosis,Follow-up and Recommendations,Events of Hospital Stay,Medications,Copies,Patient Height, Weight, BMI

Fung, Andrea Sabrina (Resident) (Signed 2017-Mar-28 15:13)

*Authored:*Goals of Care,Demographics / Care Providers,Vaccinations and Blood Products Administered,Allergies,Diagnosis,Events of Hospital Stay,Medications,Copies,Patient Height, Weight, BMI

*Entered:*Completion,Vaccinations and Blood Products Administered,Diagnosis,Follow-up and Recommendations,Events of Hospital Stay,Medications,Copies,Patient Height, Weight, BMI

Last Updated: 2017-Mar-28 15:24

Quevillon, Joey (Medical Student) (Signed 2017-Mar-24 11:26)

*Authored:*Goals of Care,Demographics / Care Providers,Vaccinations and Blood Products Administered,Allergies,Diagnosis,Follow-up and Recommendations,Events of Hospital Stay,Medications,Copies,Patient Height, Weight, BMI

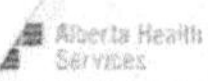

CONFIDENTIAL

Discharge Summary - Cardiac Sciences

Patient Name: **Bos, Rochelle D**   Gender: Female   Confidentiality:

RLRN: 1023394685   ULI: 866314911   Age: 70y   DOB: 1947 Jan 08   Service: Cardio

Visit/Line ID: 10004168816   Adm/Reg Date: 2017-Mar-17   Attending MD: Abdi Ali, Ahmed

Location: FMC-81-834-4

Document Created: 2017-Mar-24 By: Quevillon, Joey (Medical Student)

Medications to Continue After Discharge

Order Name	Order Summary Line
acetylsalicylic acid EC tab	81 mg PO daily
atorvastatin tab	40 mg PO qhs
nitroglycerin patch	0.4 mg/hour TOPICALLY daily at 0800h
nitroglycerin patch REMOVE	daily at 2000h
perindopril tab	2 mg PO daily
PARoxetine tab	10 mg PO daily
nitroglycerin SL spray	(Each spray delivers 0.4 mg nitroglycerin) 1 spray(s) SL q5min PRN for chest pain
bisoPROLol tab	10 mg PO daily
ezetimibe tab	10 mg PO daily
warfarin tab	(Known as: APO-WARFARIN tab) 3 mg PO once, Start at 17:00, -- Daily reassess
warfarin tab	(Known as: APO-WARFARIN tab) 3 mg PO once, Start at 17:00

Medication Reconciliation

- **Medication Reconciliation:**
  Discharge Medications are compared with the home medication list and the following changes are noted.
  Discontinued Medication and Rationale: New medications: - ASA 81mg daily - Atorvastatin 40mg qHS - Bisoprolol 10mg daily - Ezetimibe 10mg daily - Nitro patch 0.4 (daytime) - Nitro spray PRN - Perindopril 2mg daily

Family Physician Follow-up

- **Family Physician Follow-up:**
  Family physician follow-up required in one week, and the appointment will be arranged by the patient

Appointments and Referrals - Specialists

- **Primary Cardiologist:** Yes
- **Name:** Dr. Ronak Kanani
- **When:** 3 months
- **Appointment:** patient to arrange

Investigations For Physician To Arrange

- **Physician To Arrange:** Family physician

Investigations Arranged PRIOR To Discharge

- **Investigations:** Electrolytes, Creatinine
- **Result(s) to be followed up by:** Family physician

Send Copy To - Family Physician

- **Send Copy To - Family:**
  Send Copy To: Schaub, Emmanuel (Family)

Appendix F
December 2017 Discharge

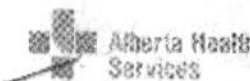

Family Doctor

CONFIDENTIAL

Discharge Summary - Cardiac Sciences

Patient Name:	Bos, Rochelle Dawn			Gender: Female	Confidentiality:
RHRN:	1023394685	ULI: 866314911	AGE: 70y	DOB: 1947-Jan-08	Service: CardSurg
Visit/Enc ID:	100045120281	Adm/Reg Date: 2017-Dec-03		Attending MD: Kidd, William Ted	
Location:	FMC-91-928-1				

Document Created 2017-Dec-04 by Krawiec, Frances (Nurse Practitioner)

Visit Data:

- Admit Date: 2017-Dec-03
- Discharge Date: 2017-Dec-24
- Discharged From: Foothills Medical Centre (FMC-91)

Goals of Care:

Goals of Care Designation R1, Designation Definition: Patient is expected to benefit from and is accepting of any appropriate investigations/interventions that can be offered including attempted resuscitation and ICU care.
This GCD has been ordered after relevant conversation with the patient. This GCD Order is unchanged from the most recent prior GCD.

Allergy and Intolerances:

Allergies:

- No Known Allergies

Cardiac Risk Factors:

- Modifiable: Dyslipidemia
- HgA1c: 5.4 % Dec 2017

History of Present Illness:

- History of Present Illness: 70 yr old lady with a history of Aortic Valve disease/BAV having two prior surgeries and last in 1997 with a mechanical AVR now presents with a history of increasing SOB and chest pain since March and two episodes of CHF. A most recent echocardiogram in August 2017 shows progression of RV/LV dysfunction including moderate RV dysfuntion, global LV shape and LVEF of 42%. The mechanical AVR is well functioning, but the patient now has severe TR. A CT chest also showed calcification in the aortic arch and descending aorta, as well as the ascending aorta is now 40mm in diameter. The patient was referred to Dr. Kidd for a redo sternotomy for tricuspid valve replacement.

At the time of surgery the patient's pacing system will be assessed for an upgrade to AV synchronization pacing.

Diagnosis:

Admitting Dx:

- Tricuspid Valve Regurgitation: Description: Tricuspid Valve Regurgitation

Past History:

- Anemia
- CHF March/May 2017
- Hemorrhoids/Polyps
- BAV

Past Surgeries:

- Remote Hand surgery
- PPM (VVIR) 2011
- Mechanical AVR 1997; Tissue AVR 1982

Diagnostic Imaging / Cardiovascular Labs:

2017-12-18 14:03, Echo Transthoracic Complete

Pertinent Lab / DI Results:

- Pertinent Lab / Diagnostic Imaging: Post op TEE - Patient had moderate LV systolic dysfunction with RWMA. Moderate RV systolic function. #28 TV annuloplasty ring insertion with mild TR. Peak gradient 3mmHg and mean gradient 1mmHg. Trace MR. All other valves were similar to pre CPB state.

COPY OF ORIGINAL	Printed From: Alberta Children's Hospital
2017-Dec-24 12:12	Job ID: 65149203
Report ID: AHS_StructuredNote_V3.rdl	Page 1 of 4

CONFIDENTIAL

Alberta Health Services

Discharge Summary - Cardiac Sciences

ent Name:	Bos, Rochelle Dawn		Gender: Female Confidentiality:
IRN:	1023394685	ULI: 866314911 AGE: 70y	DOB: 1947-Jan-08 Service: CardSurg
Visit/Enc ID:	100045120281	Adm/Reg Date: 2017-Dec-03	Attending MD: Kidd, William Ted
Location:	FMC-91-928-1		

Document Created 2017-Dec-04 by Krawiec, Frances (Nurse Practitioner)

- **Details / DI / Other:** Family MD to follow INR and dose coumadin as needed

Send Copies To:

- Kanani, Ronak Suresh (Consulting): MD-Cardiology. Active

Send Copy To - Family:

- Schaub. Emmanuel.

Send Copy To - Attending Physician:

- Kidd. William Ted (MD-Cardiac Surgery).

Send Copies to Other:

- **Other Recipients:** FMC device clinic

Completion:

- **Summary Complete**

Patient Height, Weight, BMI:

- **Weight kg:** 42.7
- **Weight was documented:** 2017-Dec-24

Blood Products Administered:

- **Blood Products Administered:** PLATELETS - Administered Doses = 1
  RED BLOOD CELLS - Administered Doses = 1

Electronic Signatures:

Krawiec. Frances **(Nurse Practitioner)** (Signed 2017-Dec-04 14:56)

Authored: Demograhics / Care Providers, Allergies, Diagnosis, Events of Hospital Stay, Follow-up and Recommendations, Copies, Patient Height, Weight, BMI

Naphin, Leisha Anne **(Nurse Practitioner)** (Signed 2017-Dec-22 16:39)

Authored: Events of Hospital Stay, Follow-up and Recommendations, Copies, Patient Height, Weight, BMI, Vaccinations and Blood Products Administered

Van Zalingen, Tracy **(Nurse Practitioner)** (Signed 2017-Dec-14 15:43)

Authored: Goals of Care, Events of Hospital Stay, Follow-up and Recommendations, Patient Height, Weight, BMI, Vaccinations and Blood Products Administered

Vetting, Ashley **(Nurse Practitioner)** (Signed 2017-Dec-24 12:12)

Authored: Demograhics / Care Providers, Diagnosis, Events of Hospital Stay, Medications, Follow-up and Recommendations, Completion, Patient Height, Weight, BMI, Vaccinations and Blood Products Administered

Last Updated: 2017-Dec-24 12:12 by Vetting. Ashley (Nurse Practitioner)

COPY OF ORIGINAL. 2017-Dec-24 12:12 Report ID: AHS_StructuredNote_V3.rdl	End of Report	Printed From: Alberta Children's Hospital Job ID: 65149203 Page 4 of 4

<table>
<tr><td>Alberta Health Services</td><td>Discharge Summary - Cardiac Sciences</td><td>CONFIDENTIAL</td></tr>
</table>

Pnt Name:	Bos, Rochelle Dawn			Gender: Female	Confidentiality:
JRN:	1023394685	ULI: 866314911	AGE: 70y	DOB: 1947-Jan-08	Service: CardSurg
Visit/Enc ID:	100045120281	Adm/Reg Date: 2017-Dec-03		Attending MD: Kidd, William Ted	
Location:	FMC-91-928-1				

Document Created 2017-Dec-04 by Krawiec, Frances (Nurse Practitioner)

Clinical Communication-Medications & IVs	, -- Goal INR: 2.5 - 3.5
enalapril tab	7.5 mg PO bid
furosemide tab	(Ordered as: LASIX tab) 40 mg PO bid 8-16
carVEDilol tab	(Ordered as: COREG tab) 3.125 mg PO bid

Medication Reconciliation:

- Discharge Medications are compared with the home medication list and the following changes are noted.
- Discontinued Medication and Rationale: Ramipril switched to Enalapril
  Bisoprolol switched to Carvedilol
  Spironolactone not resumed post op - mild AKI, to be reassessed at follow up.
- New Medications and Rationale: Pantoprazole x 6 weeks for post op GI prophylaxis
  Enalapril for severe LV dysfunction
  Carvedilol for HF/rate control

Patient Instructions:

- **Diet:** Heart Healthy; Low Sodium
- **Activity:** Gradually increasing; Sternal precautions for 6 weeks
- **Driving:** Do not drive; X 6 weeks

Family Physician Follow-up:

Family physician follow-up required in one week; Dr. Schaub and the appointment will be arranged by the patient.

Appointments and Referrals - Specialists:

- **Primary Cardiologist:** Yes
- ---> **Name:** Dr. Kanani
- ---> **When:** 2-3 months
- ---> **Appointment:** patient to arrange
- **Primary Surgeon:** Yes
- ---> **Name:** Dr. Kidd
- ---> **When:** 6-8 weeks
- ---> **Appointment:** patient to arrange

Appointments and Referrals - Clinics:

- **Cardiac Function:** Cardiac Func
- ---> **When:** TBD
- ---> **Appointment:** other doctor / office to arrange
- **Cardiac Rehabilitation:** Cardiac Rehabilitation
- ---> **When:** 1 Month
- ---> **Appointment:** Patient / Family to arrange; Referral faxed at discharge
- **Other:** Yes
- **Other Appointments and Referrals:** Device Clinic as previously arranged.
  HF clinic

Investigations Arranged PRIOR To Discharge:

- **Investigations:** INR
- **Result(s) to be followed up by:** Family physician

CONFIDENTIAL

Alberta Health
Services

Discharge Summary - Cardiac Sciences

ent Name:	**Bos, Rochelle Dawn**			Gender: Female	Confidentiality:
HRN:	1023394685	ULI: 866314911	AGE: 70y	DOB: 1947-Jan-08	Service: CardSurg
Visit/Enc ID:	100045120281	Adm/Reg Date: 2017-Dec-03		Attending MD: Kidd, William Ted	
Location:	FMC-91-928-1				

Document Created 2017-Dec-04 by Krawiec, Frances (Nurse Practitioner)

Diagnostic Imaging Special Procedures:

2017-12-21 12:50, SP Chest Tube Insertion By Rad

Surgical Procedures:

Surg Procedure:

- 2017/12/05 **Post Open Heart Reopen Bleed**. Description: 2017/12/05 Post Open Heart Reopen Bleed
- 2017/12/05 **Redo Redo Sternotomy; Tricuspid Valve Replacement**. Description: 2017/12/05 Redo Redo Sternotomy; Tricuspid Valve Replacement

Surgical Procedures:

- Cardiac Resynchronization Therapy 2017-Dec-05. Medtronic Consulta CRT-P-C3
  Medtronic Atrial lead 4968 CapSure-Epi
  RV Greatbatch 511212, SN 267876
  LV Greatbatch 511212 SN 252506.
- Tricuspid Valve 2017-Dec-05. Edwards Lifesciences Ring size 28 mm.

Complications:

- Acute Renal Failure; Atrial Fibrillation: Heart Failure.

Course In Hospital:

Complicated OR for bleeding chest left open. Closed on POD #1

CVICU complicated by
1. Prolonged ventilation likely secondary to heart failure and post op atelectasis, self extubated POD # 8 to bipap

2. Atrial fibrillation - treated with amiodarone load. Paced at time of transfer to ward. OAC for mechanical AVR

3. Dysphagia - cleared by SLP December 14. Normal oral pharyngeal swallow

Other post operative issues
1. Volume overload in the setting of biventricular dysfunction - followed by the Advanced heart failure team
for optimization of medical therapies. Will need ongoing outpatient follow up to be arranged by Heart failure liaison nurse.

2. Left pleural effusion - chest tube insertion for 1.2L over 48H. Removed Dec 23/17. Follow up CXR showed small residual left pleural
effusion and tiny right effusion.

3. UTI - Treated with a 7 day course of ciprofloxacin

4. Mild AKI - improving at time of discharge

Medications:

Medications to Continue After Discharge:

ORDER NAME	ORDER SUMMARY LINE
atorvastatin tab	(Ordered as: LIPITOR tab) 40 mg PO qhs
PARoxetine tab	10 mg PO daily
pantoprazole EC tab	40 mg PO daily before breakfast. --Discharge Reminder: The current lowest cost PPI has been used in hospital. Patient's home medication may differ.
acetylsalicylic acid EC tab	(Ordered as: ASA EC tab) 81 mg PO daily
zopiclone tab	5 mg PO qhs PRN
Clinical Communication-Medications & IVs	, -- Daily warfarin dosing

www.ingramcontent.com/pod-product-compliance
Lightning Source LLC
Chambersburg PA
CBHW070717250726
48662CB00001B/465